Sacred Choices

Numinous Publishing

Sacred Choices

accessing the astrology of our celestial overlay

patricia phillips

Numinous Publishing

pO Box 2063

sedona, arizona 86339-2063

928-634-1345

Copyright © 2010 by Numinous Publishing

Cover art by patricia phillips

Cover, text design and layout by matthew simons and patricia phillips

ISBN: 978-0-9764352-2-8

All rights reserved. Printed in the United States of America.

Please enjoy. . . .

Copyright © 2010 Numinous Publishing

Thanks is gratefully extended to the following publishers and authors for permission to reprint excerpts:

from *The Book of Sound Therapy* by Olivea Dewhurst-Maddock. Used with permission from N.Y. Simon & Schuster, copyright © 1993.

from *The Lost Language of Plants* by Stephen Harrod Buhner, copyright © 2002. Used with permission from Chelsea Green Publishing Co., White River Junction, Vermont (www.chelseagreen.com).

from *In Search of the Medicine Buddha* by David Crow, copyright © 2000 by David Crow. Used by permission of Jeremy P. Tarcher, an imprint of Penguin Group (USA) Inc.

from *Tachyon Energy: A New Paradigm in Holistic Healing* by David Wagner and Gabriel Cousens, published by North Atlantic Books, copyright © 1999 by Gabriel Cousens and David Wagner. Reprinted by permission of publisher.

from *Spiritual Nutrition and the Rainbow Diet* by Gabriel Cousens, published by Cassandra Press, copyright © 1986 by Gabriel Cousens. Reprinted by permission of author.

from *Earth in Ascension* by Nancy Ann Clark, copyright © 1995 Nancy Ann Clark. Used with permission from Nancy Ann Clark and Violet Fire Publishing.

from *Return of the Children of Light* by Judith Bluestone Polich, copyright © 2001 Judith Bluestone Polich. Used with permission from Bear & Company, Rochester, Vermont (www.innertraditions.com).

from *Spiritual Alchemy: How To Transform Your Life* by Dr. Christine Page, published by Rider with C. W. Daniel. Reprinted by permission of The Random House Group Ltd.

from *Sacred Geometry: Philosophy and Practice* by Robert Lawlor. Used with permission from N.Y. Thames & Hudson Inc., copyright © 1982.

from *Energy Blessings from the Stars: Seven Initiations* by Irving Feurst & Virginia Essene, copyright © 1998 Irving Feurst. Used with permission from Spiritual Education Endeavors Publishing Co.

from *You Are Becoming A Galactic Human* by Virginia Essene & Sheldon Nidle, copyright © 1994 Virginia Essene & Sheldon Nidle. Used with permission from Spiritual Education Endeavors Publishing Co.

from *New Cells, New Bodies, New Life!* by Virginia Essene, copyright © 1991 Virginia Essene. Used with permission from Spiritual Education Endeavors Publishing Co.

with love and compassion

as we move forward on our sacred journeys

abbreviating a catalogue of gratitude

In reflecting back across the years during which this volume was birthing, as well as back across the months and weeks during which it has so recently birthed, I am moved with gratitude and humility by the tapestry of Spirit's synchronicities that has made Sacred Choices possible.

Returning from such a reflective meditation, I would like to thank my dearly loved college roommate and grade-school friend, Ann, for her love and patience, her acceptance and encouragement, for her grace, her refinement, and her sensitivity over these nearly five decades — and especially for the elixir of her laughter and her wondrous sense of humour and for that phone chat one October or November morning when she suggested with all sincerity that I should write this book.

And my most loving thanks to Leslie and Brian for warmly welcoming me into their family and indeed for becoming mine, replete with dogs and goats, pheasants and guineas, rabbits and horses, and the possibilities of peacocks and llamas in the future; and additionally for building next door their dreamhouse-in-the-country and inviting me to share in the growing-up adventures of two enchanting little souls.

Michele, dear one, thank you for the magic of our connection in design and metaphysics and for being my treasured psychic partner in dowsing and in the sharing of psycho-spiritual texts, seminars, experiencings, and observations.

Reverend Zemke and Leslee, thank you for your intuitive wisdom, your love and your seamless connection both with Source and with your Sacred Guidance and for softening the blessing opportunities of my incarnation by positioning them in the purposefulness and future consciousness of their celestial parameters.

And Kyle, thank you for your endless patience and good spirits, blessing consistently my queasiness about deadlines and typefaces with your calm and endless reassurance. Thank you, too, for the exquisite gift of your computer and graphics skill sets and so much for monitoring the transformation of my post-it trimmed manuscript into a choreography of dimensionality and nuance.

And indeed my deepest appreciation, Rick, for your kindness and your extraordinary printing skills and for your incredible commitment and loving attentiveness to each delicate nuance and detail as you have shepherded Sacred Choices from the cyber realms of pdf into the turnable pages of printed copy from which I've been so more happily able to edit.

And thank you blessing and synchronistic universe for overseeing the attracting in of friends and friends of friends to support my efforts and my extreme need and vulnerability when my design team has unexpectedly been drawn to resign and I've felt increasingly and unalterably the approaching dates of copyright permission deadlines. Thank you Janet and Cliff for guiding me with such kindness and focused choices and reassurances when my own compass has felt anything but stable.

Nancy, my gratitude and my delight in our editing hours together know no boundaries, and it has surely been under your professorial eye that Sacred Choices has strengthened in grammar and construction.

Marianna, your warmth, your enthusiasm, and your deliciously infectious and upbeat spirit have honoured our project in the ultimate sense — inspiring trust and offering promise and reassurance. Your wonderful energy combined with your computer wizardry and eagerness to work most effectively and efficiently in tandem with our new graphics and layout designer have made possible a fully corrected manuscript, ready in every discoverable typo and footnoted nuance to assume her publishable presence.

And Matt, under your caring supervision and with parameterless patience, your blessing skills and the refinement and the sensitivity of your inner vision have birthed Sacred Choices in a subtle wardrobe of fonts and bejeweled her with the visual rhythms (and the occasional counterpoint) of leadings and margins, point sizes and screens.

Sacred Choices has clearly found a loving home with Numinous Publishing where Lin David, my friend and mentor from our years in Sedona with his bride, Torill, direct this splendid tool of spiritual communication and confirmation. Dear Torill, your patience, your vision, and your encouragement have been invaluable. You've resolved detail after detail with seemingly endless receptivity and quietly, with focus on fluidity and the interconnectivity of its voice, you have evoked a text with inner structure and inherent amplitude for completing the vision of optimism and possibility it proclaims.

In looking inside with quiet intent, it feels clear that there has only ever been this one research-inclusive volume in my heart — this metaphysically conscious collectivity dancing around the possibilities of health and nature and galactic evolution. So many shapes she might have embraced, only now having birthed herself as <u>Sacred Choices</u>, she feels content — willing to let those next aspects of herself birth in the minds of those who read her and in their exchanges with volumes suggested as supplemental and potentially supportive. Skimming back across a history of emotion and spiritual intent, I'm drawn to expand this litany of gratitude to thank those belovéd ones who have so profoundly touched my life and shared in shaping the synchronicities of her psychological architecture. I would thus seek your understanding in the paragraphs that follow and/or just as sincerely encourage you to hopscotch beyond them into the body of the text if that appeals more.

First, I want to thank my father who has always encouraged his children to embrace their spiritual understandings as they have seemed most clear for them, notwithstanding or limited in any way by his own profound immersion in Episcopal doctrine as the highly evolved Initiate that he is. And I want to thank him for his treasured gift in honour of my ordination, namely a pencil slim, greiged, water-blue Bible of my choosing with a message of his love inscribed in the frontispiece.

I want also to thank Father Taliaferro, an Episcopal priest and Rosicrucian master and my father's best friend, under whose loving wisdom and guidance I began my spiritual studies in this incarnation, working in tandem with the Rosicrucian monographs and the Alice Bailey volumes — those treasured mid-twentieth century treatises received from the Tibetan Master, Djwhal Khul.

Also my mother, for the loving breadth of her introduction to the magics of color, music, and nature; for her tenderness manifesting equally with Chopin, fledglings and ocelots; and so especially for the model of selflessness and unlimited generosity and empathy she lived.

And my Aunt Susan who introduced me to the esoteric theatres of astrology and to her friend Dane Rudhyar.

Ingrid Stadler, the sparkly-eyed chair of the philosophy department at Wellesley in 1970, who encouraged me with love and wisdom in my request to visually design my final philosophy papers addressing Sartre's <u>Nausea</u> and Wittgenstein's "private language argument" respectively.

My sister, Spin, for her patience, her love and her acceptance, and so especially for her honesty and caring integrity in sharing with me on many occasions her profound and truly guiding observations.

My sister, Kalita, for her beautiful and non-judgmental wisdom and for all the magics of discovering that one's little sister loves her older sister.

My brother, Peter, whose soft spoken both/and embrace of life and her challenges evokes such respect and such trust.

Our knowing friend, Roger, Hermetic astrologer and patient prof., whose wisdom and quiet clarity has so enhanced my work and with whom I've spent so many profound and inwardly clarifying hours considering the journey of the soul and positioning her in the framework of her celestial birthchart.

My treasured friend Janet whose visionary and intuitive gifts have blessed my wobblings again and again with affirmation and expanded interpretations.

And I want to thank Robert for introducing me to the blessing wisdoms of terrain, polarity, morbidity, and the Life Force connecting qualities of the cerebral spinal fluid throughout the body and for teaching me to observe, to honour, and to aid our bodies in their profound ableness to heal themselves by offering them those bits of information that they can best use to return to balance. I also want to thank you, Robert, for giving so deeply of yourself in sharing your radionic knowingness with your students and your inspired esoteric and exoteric embrace of simplicity and its application to Malcolm Rae's system as you interpreted it *for* us and taught it *to* us.

And Barry and Audre, thank you for your love and your patience in opening for me the devic realms engaged with Nature's gift of her essential oils. Thank you for untangling the limitations of my earlier understandings so that I could link the joys of my devic and fairy friendships with the oils and with the blessing privilege

abbreviating a catalogue of gratitude

of honouring and encouraging our bodies in their efforts to re-embrace their interpretation of balance.

And still there is so much more to be thankful for — indeed for life itself and the blessing choice of being here at this time. And gratitude too for so many other loving souls whose smiles and questions and committed pursuit of their spiritual journeys have so blessed my own.

Notwithstanding, let me draw these thoughts to a conclusion in thanking my belovéd husband, Charles, who throughout our twenty years together has so profoundly blessed my life with sixth and seventh dimensional opportunities that I hesitate to believe I could or would have embraced for myself with the same quantum depth of interior learning and self-observation. And thank you as well, dear one, for introducing me with reverence and wonderment to the resonant interaction of your ants and bees with their respective worlds, to the vibratory beckoning of the flowers and their families of insects, to the auras of cacti and crystals, and to the electromagnetics and the sentiency of the human anatomy, and perhaps most of all for introducing me to those shamanic realms of the sacred and ritualistic grace of consciousness in expansion.

a guide to information included

honouring us all as we journey forward	*ix*
abbreviating a catalogue of gratitude	*xi*
a guide to information included	*xvii*
a publisher's foreword	*xxiii*
a few gentle questions	*xxv*

part the first: options

i	introducing parameters of embrace	*39*
ii	unsettling our pessimisms	*45*
iii	moving in tandem across an evolving landscape	*51*
iv	moving through our fears and our fear-based beliefs into places of trust	*55*
v	observing the glorious neutrality of *is, allness, wholeness, and I am that I am* dawning in humanity's evolving consciousness	*61*
vi	honouring our cosmic role as a brilliant planetary experiment of grace and sentiency	*65*

vii	outsourcing cause and the affective continuity of our thoughts and feelings	69
viii	attracting health, reviewing our interior landscape, and unveiling a future beyond spiritual amnesia	73

part the second: blessings

ix	marveling at Nature's innate wisdom	81
x	identifying frequencies and Nature's energetic blessings	87
xi	inviting possibilities and partnering with Nature	95

part the third: appendices
an annotated anthology

sketching a dream of fluidity and trust: revelations of life unveiling beyond limitation and fear	111
Appendix A: excerpts from <u>The Lost Language of Plants</u>	115
Appendix B: excerpts from <u>In Search of the Medicine Buddha</u>	133
Appendix C: excerpts from <u>Tachyon Energy</u>	141
Appendix D: excerpts from <u>Earth in Ascension</u>	147
Appendix E: excerpts from <u>Return of the Children of Light</u>	161
Appendix F: excerpts from <u>Energy Blessings from the Stars</u>	183
Appendix G: excerpts from <u>You Are Becoming a Galactic Human</u>	195
Appendix H: transcription of a ***corridor*** meditation	227

part the fourth: sources cited

    celebrating guidance, abundance and
    life-altering thoughts

    books   *237*

    courses, discussions, and seminars   *238*

part the fifth: supplementary readings and visuals
    a celebration of options

    sketching again: visions of forward
    and the sacrement of choice   *245*

    earth's energies and sacred sites and geometries   *247*

    the *new* energy   *248*

    the Shift   *250*

    esoteric Christianity   *251*

    reincarnation   *254*

    unfolding the cosmic tapestry   *256*

    children   *261*

    intuition   *262*

    inspiration   *263*

    angels and guides   *264*

    shamanism   *265*

entheogens	267
animals	267
nature	268
wicca	269
psychological health	270
health	276
healers	278
supplements (primarily from plants)	279
alternative modalities	280
gems and crystals	282
dowsing	283
runes	283
numerology	283
music	284
aromatherapy	286

part the sixth: showcasing the future

affirming simplicty and the grace of conciousness in expansion	
publications	293
future focused organizations	293

publisher's foreword

Sacred Choices: accessing the astrology of our celestial overlay, developed from a five-page assignment on the future role of Medicinal Aromatherapy into an in-depth look at the expansion of human consciousness and the use of different healing modalities — including Medicinal Aromatherapy — to aid us humans in this process of waking up to a greater reality.

What a grand challenge to take on — and Phillips impressively completes the task with success and grace because of her greater understanding and ability to translate knowingness into delightful reading.

To supply the reader with a broad spectrum of insights available to us at this point in time, Phillips includes an *annotated anthology* (page 107) of enlightening material from many different sources, in addition to a rich *supplementary reading* list (page 241).

As she is sharing in *a celebration of options* (page 245): "I am hopeful that the excerpts you have just read can serve as shortcuts and as possible tools for locating further readings in case any of those included have evoked greater interest or an etheric connection of resonant response."

Seldom do you find this many evolved teachings collected in the same volume. We thank you Patricia for building golden bridges between seemingly disparate viewpoints and showing us that they all have their place and that they all point in the same direction — towards a more holistic perception and understanding.

a few gentle questions

Could we position an overview of medicinal aromatherapy's role in our future amidst quiltings of galactic historical contexts (past and present) interwoven and overwoven with spider strands of non-fear and of that glorious elasticity of possibility and anticipation?

Could we choose to emphasize the role of human thought and emotion as those continuous self-giftings having greater impact on our health, and on our blessed planet's health than all else combined – indeed the bipartite domain from which heralds most cause and most effect?

Do we know well enough the value of looking out at life on our planet without fear and without judgment from the umbrellaed protection of understanding galactic pasts and futures?

Indeed, do we notice our attitude and the quality of our joy in seeking for the perfection in all and in responding to non-peace by being peace?*

* *Audre Wenzler Guttierez, my dear friend and teacher, first introduced me to this thought.*

if our thoughts, actions

and responses are all embraced with

love and compassion and with

the non-fear of knowing the assuaging peace

of the incarnational cycle and the blessing

of the cyclical timbre of death,

then it is not usually necessary

to be unwell

may we listen both with our souls

and to our souls as we remember who we are and

as we re-awaken to the divinity in ourselves

and in the oils

the ensuing pages intend to paint with

the wisdom of integrating options

part the first:

———

options

introducing parameters of embrace | *i*

The elastic and breathing parameters of the role of medicinal aromatherapy in and into the future have encouraged me to reformat the academic paper initially prepared for an advanced seminar and from which has been crafted the pages of the volume you now hold. Areas of consideration span past, present, and future tenses — cosmologies of indigenous cultures and dictées of galactic purposefulness and intentionality — ecologies subsiding, and ecosystems in disarray . . .

co-creative gardening with devic intelligence . . .

embracing the wizardry of tachyon energies and subtle organizing energy fields for the blessing and healing of humanity's consciousness of herself . . .

observing the increasing morbidity of all that we can't digest, whether physically, emotionally, mentally, or spiritually; and into all of this, the giftlessness of antibiotics and the mainstream pursuit of symptoms as causes . . .

and finally, delineating causation's link with our thoughts and feelings and indeed with our mental and emotional subtle bodies and the energetic match we must be to welcome in the frequency and the wake-up calling quality of the events in our lives and of the diseases we think we contract . . .

Indeed with such an expansive content to be reviewed, I've chosen to offer a collection of thoughts on healing options and opportunities as we approach our individual human and collective planetary futures, followed by extended excerpts from seven volumes in the form of appendices. Introductory comments reflect or facet in some manner my responses to the materials included, and one final appendix unfolds in the form of a transcription — a sequential collection of nuances and symbols cataloguing my participation in a ***corridor*** meditation of self-discovery. In conclusion, I've offered a syllabus of selected readings that more deeply acquaints us with a galactic continuum of events (tripartite histories through possible and intended futures), a causative embrace of health and healing, and an unveiling of the energetic and psycho-spiritual blessings of unconditional love and unconditional compassion.

At first I struggled to find a seamless transition and orderliness with unrepeated information for the collection of pages that have emerged over these last weeks as I've set about addressing the role of aromatherapy both in the future and in our future as human beings (even if we may well be spiritual beings having some of our pre-chosen

human experiences). And then in the twinkling of an eye, in response to my asking (after two or three self-directed days of struggle with reading and re-reading these pages), my treasured angel presences slipped into my consciousness a truly delicious resolution to my increasing trauma — "Just include them all. They've all come from your heart — snatches from 5 a.m.s and 2 a.m.s as well as midnights and late mornings . . . we ask you to trust that in their seeming redundance lies exactly their effect. Their repetition will simply serve to reinforce that which you hold so preciously true — the *boths* and *ands* and the exquisite details and nuances of those same *boths* and *ands* that further celebrate the dawning of a sixth dimensional paradigm." So with what feels for me an angelic gift of sanction for this journaled-style, join me in considering the blessings of medicinal aromatherapy in our respective futures.

unsettling our pessimisms

As it sinks in that we are spiritual beings created in God's image, blessed with a divine spark — indeed each of us a droplet in the same ocean we call divinity — and each of us having come both to learn and to serve, we are changed. Just a belief of such skeletal simplicity could release us to participate with love, patience, wisdom, and gratitude unperturbed by the human competitions and dramas we've been used to arranging for ourselves both interiorly and exteriorly with co-workers and family members, etc.

Scholastic laddering, corporate laddering, and laddering up the social fabric of our communities are the masquerades we've been drawn to repeat in the social landscape of daily living. A subtle one-upping malgraces our participation in the classroom and later in the boardroom and later still in those group settings clustered around a sport or an activity, a charity or a belief system, religious or otherwise. And where are we anyway when we arrive at these hypothetical zeniths? And what if we could relax — relax into our own joy and interior safety instead? What if winning weren't the issue? What if my success were also your success? And what if we could only succeed? — what if failure weren't an option? — and the whole concept simply ceased to exist? What if we moved into that knowingness that it never had existed and never could exist except by fabrication in the minds of men attuned to an *illusion* of power held rigorously in place by the cognoscenti and the god-mongering of their priests and parochial mentors? Indeed, what if we relaxed into the blessing and the privilege of being alive — what if we could let ourselves choose a line of pursuit for which we actually felt passion — or could allow our life to be about joy — or even to be that joy rather than about that joy? What if there were an inner terrain of such peace and self-knowing, co-existing with such a profound joyfulness that less than smooth patches were embraced with understanding and trust and unable to jostle that inner peace? It wouldn't have to mean, belovéd ones, that these pockets of lesser smooth were unrealistically wanded away — fairy godmother style — just that our relationship with them could shift from harmonics of dread and fear into harmonies of self-knowing, acceptance, and gratitude. And it could also mean that we would newly honour these lows for the synchronistic gifts and wake-up nudges they so really can be allowed to become. They can make potentially available to us whole next levels of relationship with ourselves and with our friends and family members and indeed with the very incarnation in question and with how we're mirroring it both *to* and *for* ourselves.

Protecting and honouring our planet's ecosystems is certainly critical, but can we really best participate or serve in groups toward this end before we can access our

own inner peace? Bringing a quiet inward knowingness to the global endeavour of shifting the consciousness of the human family seems our link with flowing into and through 2012's glorious gift of the Ages Shifting. Two nuances emerge in reviewing the above: First, that it seems to be about living harmoniously, i.e., in generic harmony *with* or generically *in* harmony with, and second, that as profound frequency-shifts in our inner beings reach critical mass, the planet and the rest of the human family shift also.

If the appendices in Sacred Choices can in any way increase our inner assuagedness and mitigate our ableness and/or need to worry quite so extensively — if Sacred Choices can have made it possible for even one person to feel less entangled with unknowns he's not yet been able to wrap his career or his spiritual life around, then it will have honoured successfully the intention that has spawned it. This anthology-style collectivity of others' thoughts, stretching in its lengthy discursive style to engage readers long enough and with sufficient interest in areas they may not yet have consciously considered, intends to unsettle their pessimisms and their marriages with finite worlds of seeable and provable.

*moving in tandem
across an evolving landscape*

It is so important that we do not further terrorize people who are already troubled by the current tenses of lives they often experience as verging on out-of-control. People having a semi-openness *to* or semi-awareness *of* the esoteric will be those most especially concerned by echoes they hear about the conclusion of the Mayan Calendar and about any number of other shoulds, oughts, and possibilities they overhear from more esoterically clear and energetically aware persons. Shoulds and oughts about *raising one's frequency* and about critical aftermaths for those who are not able to or do not choose to are all the more complicated when a phrase like *raising one's frequency* may not even be a familiar term. So much fear is nurtured on our planet at this time and not just by the everyday societal disturbances of finances, health, job security, emotional and familial instabilities, etc.[1] but equally, if not more so, by spiritual and New Age concepts and confusions verbally bandied about. And there is also a growing alarm in finding that the spiritual understandings of orthodox religions no longer advise or as meaningfully or appropriately answer the needs and issues of parishioners and communicants. Everyday issues assigned dogmatic interpretations simply don't assuage any longer.

Looking out over vistas of humanity's potential futures, it doesn't appear to me that suggesting medicinal aromatherapy as our primary tool for serving humanity's health needs corresponds sufficiently with what we believe we know about humanity and planet Earth moving in tandem across an evolving landscape toward multi-dimensionality and exquisitely higher frequencies. Into such a setting I would rather want to introduce self-knowledge and an underlying sense of purposefulness, both critical as we address the terrain of our health, and both areas to which the devic wisdom of aromatherapy's astounding capacity can and does contribute profoundly. Into this bouillabaisse of tools I would also add an awareness of the extraordinary gift of tachyon energies and the regulatory properties of our subtle organizing energy fields (SOEFS) along with an increasing familiarity with Earth's galactic history and potential future. I think these areas of focus would serve us very well indeed, as would a more meaningful and functional understanding of the link between our health and our emotions, our feelings, our thoughts, and our thoughts' patterns — for they constitute a medicine with which we treat ourselves continuously and without the capacity for pause. Ultimately, gifting ourselves with the upper register frequencies of unconditional love and unconditional compassion is where I'd lovingly anchor the energetics of both my diagnostic and my prognostic efforts for mankind.

---

[1] Indeed a time when the earlier social matterfulness of the prominence or non-prominence of our families of origin or where we went to school just doesn't hold the same weight.

*moving through our fears and
our fear-based beliefs into places of trust* | *iv*

Suggesting that medicinal aromatherapy could be the primary healing modality should our planet undergo cataclysmic changes in connection with the Shift of the Ages synchronized with the conclusion of the Mayan calendar in December of 2012, gives pause for several reflections.[2] First of all, I hold dear a belief in a profound and inner shift in frequency and in consciousness that even in the most dire of scenarios would still soften the edges of whatever physically, geographically, and/or anatomically manifests in conjunction with the above mentioned Shift of 2012.[3] Furthermore, I am persuaded that humanity's collective and individual healing will come from this shift in consciousness and from a dawning awareness of purpose and meaning both on the planet and as part of our galactic unity. Moving through our fears and our fear-based beliefs into places of trust seems profoundly medicinal on all planes — physical, emotional, mental, and spiritual. And as the veils between the dimensions become thinner and more diaphanous, certainly it will be in this energetic repositioning of our emotional and psycho-spiritual assemblage points that much of the inner homework will need to be done, although there is no doubt that it can be exquisitely nurtured and supported by the devic gifts of the essential oils. Many would suggest (and I certainly concur) that the oils in being invoked to help with these shifts in consciousness can support them both as they are shifting and as the shifts are being anchored in.

All the same, it feels as though an introduction to our galactic and planetary history and intended futures can fundamentally shift both our focus and our intention as can Henry Lindlahr's introduction to his <u>Philosophy</u> of <u>Natural</u> <u>Therapeutics</u> shift our understanding *of* and subsequent response *to* cause and effect's manifestation as disease in the physical body. Lindlahr's impact and capacity for shifting our point of view parallels the convincing pedagogy of David Crow in his <u>In</u> <u>Search</u> <u>of</u> <u>the</u> <u>Medicine</u> <u>Buddha</u>, of Stephen Buhner in his Lost Language of Plants, and of Gregg Braden in his <u>Walking</u> <u>Between</u> <u>the</u> <u>Worlds</u>.[4-5]

As we come to know the emotional and psycho-spiritual ability to relax into the acceptance of ourselves as the quintessence of our vibratory offering (albeit achieved, evolved and tweaked along the journey of our experiencings), then we can begin, in a

---

[2] I so don't want to further invoke fear that even just placing my consciousness here for long enough to write *cataclysmic* comes perilously close to violating my sense of what could serve humanity better at this critical time.

[3] By which I'm really wanting to suggest that I believe the Shift is likely to be a predominantly inner one (at all levels of our physical and subtle anatomies) or that at least with humanity's helping efforts it can be

[4] Please see *Appendices D, E, F,* and *G*.

[5] Please see *Sources Cited* for complete publishing details on the texts cited.

major way, to nurture our belovéd selves with the medicinal and energetic continuity of our self-love and our universal compassion. The huge stress of defining ourselves by our achievements lends an image of endless treadmilling devoid of the inner relaxation and self-acceptance earlier sketched.[6]

---

[6] Where relaxation is not alluding to a goal-free existence of idyllic joblessness — rather an inner state of relaxation — valuing time to rejoice in life and nature — and in using those gifts we each have to honour that purpose for which we believe we've chosen our current incarnation here on Earth just prior to her Shift.

*observing the glorious neutrality of **is, all-ness, wholeness,** and **I am that I am** dawning in humanity's evolving consciousness*

Many healing modalities will serve humanity as she evolves and will serve specific individuals as they find themselves in resonance *with* or through resonance drawn *to* particular healing modalities by an esoteric magnetism based on an earlier familiarity with them bleeding through, if you will, from previous timeframes in their incarnational heritage.

If tachyon awarenesses resonate with 'q,'[7] it seems logical that 'q's' energetic and virtually unsought knowledge of tachyon merit and matterfulness on a universal scale as well as on a personal scale, in the unique paradigm of being 'q,' should be both profoundly honoured and as profoundly embraced. It can be safely assumed that the use of such tachyon energies in all aspects of 'q's' transformative process can and will be compelling. By contrast, even to suggest that honouring the vast wisdom and healing ableness of Mother Earth's devic gifts (in the context of her essential oils) would be a valid first choice and a better healing choice for 'q' and for the planet in the case of 'q,' seems to lack flexibility and overview. Emphasizing either/or applies the same duality to our planet's original healing modality that we are striving so pointedly to move beyond as a race and as a family. It is rather a time for expansiveness and for emphasizing *both* and *and* as we transition and transform from this consciousness of duality into one of unity — where all forms of erstwhile dual perception can be cradled in the omniversal awareness of a unity in which they are all part of one another as we are of each other. Let us note that in almost every case, the assignation of positive and negative values has come from our human orientation while the glorious neutrality of *Is, All-ness, Wholeness,* and *I Am that I Am* that begins to dawn in humanity's evolving and unveiling consciousness, moves ahead without the emotional weight of its erstwhile egoic component.

---

[7] 'q' represents a hypothetical person for the sake of the text.

*honouring our cosmic role as a brilliant
planetary experiment of grace and sentiency*

Even at the risk of repetition, let me reiterate that to heal as human beings and as a planet, an awareness of our incarnational history and of our incarnational and galactic future is of profound importance. Equally, as a race we have a great need to be more accurately informed in three areas: first, how health is generated; second, where causality fits in its relationship with health; and third, but as a subheading under causality, a need to consider the affective continuity (be it nourishing or poisonous) of something as elemental as the quality of our thoughts and the quality of our emotions. I do not wish to have written solely for the sake of honouring an academic trust. I have preferred instead to create a body of references in addition to honouring the general theme of the future of medicinal aromatherapy so that I (and others too) can use this work as a reference tool for further study and further evolution of our understanding of Mother Nature and of our cosmic role as a brilliant planetary experiment of grace and sentiency in the galactic order of this universe and others.

outsourcing cause and the affective continuity of our thoughts and feelings

There is an inner peace, a vibrational harmony and a shifting frequency conceptually linked with feeling more familiar with our own history and potential future. One can then be less traumatized by the hearsay of anatomical and geographic catastrophes anticipated as an accompaniment to the closing of the Mayan calendar. Before we can choose aromatherapy as our loving guide, perhaps we should truly understand from whence disease and physical disharmony herald — indeed from whence they are sourced and to what allopathy has allocated cause. And it is key to note that even with aromatherapy's nurturing ableness to shift the quality of our thoughts and outlook without our direct intention or wakeful consciousness of it, if we are not consciously able to grasp which thought forms and thought patterns have welcomed in or magnetically attracted in which disease and which whys are supporting it's particular degree of severity, then however able the oils have been in helping it to depart, it will return again as a blessing wake-up call in direct ratio and intensity with the qualitative rutted-outness of our thoughts and our emotional patterns. As first aid and loving nurturer, as supplement to our inflammations, burns, bruises, cuts, and depressions, etc., aromatherapy can be of extraordinary support. And yet, even here we are best served to know deeper into causation, as nothing is by chance, be it a cut finger or a torn ligament. Each will have been attracted to that body part or area for exactly that right reason — magnetized exactly there for all the wise reasons that underlie every seeming *by chance* and where *by chance* is always the blessing gift of synchronicity. As we evolve, we are inwardly encouraged or prompted perhaps to let the veil of coincidence lift upon the diaphanous and beautiful mindscape of synchronicity. Increasingly, details assume roles of consequence as symbols in the personal solarium of our intuition's blossoming, and we find ourselves embracing with far greater appreciation and understanding that hypothetical meditation so often serving in sessions and seminars of self-discovery — the one asking: who are you as you move down your **corridor** towards the door through which you must pass to arrive on the other side? Indeed, who are you and what symbols are revealed and created to share their meaning with you as you verbally sketch your **corridor**, your door, and your *what's-on-the-other-side?*[8]

---

[8] Please see *Appendix H*.

attracting health
reviewing our interior landscape
and unveiling a future beyond spiritual amnesia

attracting health and reviewing our interior landscape

There are those among us who will wish to pursue their greater health down avenues of psychological self-remembrance, others who will most resonate with sound[9] in their efforts to remember who they are and why they are here, and still others who will be as unequivocally drawn to colour, space, and light[10] in their sacred quest for self-rememberfulness. And in the end, with all things equally and fairly considered, is not good health sourced from self-knowledge, self-love, and that self-awareness that has come to remember why we've chosen planet Earth in this very particular timeframe and what we've intended to learn and how we've intended to serve during our sojourn here (referencing the current incarnation)? Included here must be the inner attitude of our response to the given incarnation and to our understanding of the cosmos and of our place and our planet's place in it. With the imperative of focusing on who we are and why we are here can surface the cardinal realization that disease is often — perhaps even most often — a manifestation of the pursuit of our personality's path rather than our soul's — and certainly our bodies will always ultimately honour and serve the soul over the personality (Page, *Level 1 Seminar*). The quintessential frequency and difference of loving or of somehow losing ourselves in fears cleverly name-tagged with all those acceptable *reasons why*, is key in the magnetization process of attracting in health or lesser health. Our bodies never fail to know how we really feel and over time can bless us with the wake-up calls of cysts

---

[9] It is said that we have each a keynote which in simply hearing for some of us seems almost to open worlds orgasmically. It can be played for almost however short a period — just that during that time the ethers must be as if suffused with the frequency of the given tone e.g., so that for however brief a time, the texture will still be far more complete, far more dense, than the audibly sheerer texture of a staccato or pizzicato address or attack of the same temporal duration on this sacred note we're highlighting. (It is the key of 'e' that so enchants my incarnation in this fairytale style and especially when offered on the E♭ clarinet). Let me draw these thoughts together in adding several further observations about sound — quoting from Oliver Dewhurst-Maddock's Book of Sound Therapy where she suggests that:

"Human consciousness presently roams between two vibratory parameters: the life-span of the universe, and the minutest vibration of an atom. The long-sought fulcrum or balance point is elusive, being hidden within the itinerant soul or spirit of ourselves. Beyond the physical body and the intellectual self-knowing mind, the most significant therapeutic expansion is that of identity: 'Who am I?' Living organisms exist within physically and biologically defined structures, but our human consciousness has no such boundaries. Enlightenment and healing are achieved by the extension of our vibratory spectrum, inward to our emotions and hearts, and out to the planet, Gaia, and ultimately to the cosmos.

Healing relies on an openness to the whole; a willingness to relinquish whatever frustrates or delays — mistaken ideas, negative feelings, poor diet, inadvisable lifestyle — and to accept a wider spectrum of responses with new ideas, experiences, and priorities. Healing is communication; and music, in its universal nature, is total communication. In the deepest mysteries of music are the inspirations, the pathways, and the healing which lead to one-ness and unity." (Dewhurst-Maddock 120-121)

[10] Consider for example someone coming from star systems where the diaphanous beauty of light is all-engaging and for whom there is therefore self-remembering in the delicate mauves and aquas of bubble baths and dragonfly wings married with the emotional magic of pre-storm drama, clarity, cool and light.

and cancers and other dis-eases in an effort to provide the guidance that can capture our attention. With our greatest attentiveness, if we could accord ourselves even a microfissure of self-love and self-acceptance unblemished with fear, it could allow us to honestly review our interior landscapes however devoid of joy and of enthusiasm we might have to notice that they are at this time. Spiritual amnesia is perhaps the malady of note in the Christian world. It has blessed us for centuries in our efforts to learn through challenges — indeed through challenges and dramas from whose purposefulness we've felt excluded and yet without which the learnings made available from said challenges wouldn't have been available for us. Now, though, as we transcend our three-dimensional polarity-based paradigm into the initiations of the fifth dimension, amnesia no longer serves the same purpose and she is receding in favour of unconditional love and compassion and the inclusiveness of a both/and paradigm.

part the second:

---

blessings

marveling at Nature's innate wisdom

marveling at Nature's innate wisdom

The range of blessings and gifts from our belovéd friends the trees and the plants to our planet and to humanity exceeds bountifully even our keenest imaginations. Those of us who are not ecologists, biologists, ethnobotanists, or ecosystem analysts or otherwise similarly engaged, may well be astounded by the delicate nuances of Nature's innate knowingness and the phenomenal details of those life-generating systems in which she participates and to which she contributes in just the creationing of our atmosphere.

Stephen Buhner, in his Lost Language of Plants, introduces us again and again to the magnitude of Nature, both as a global ecosystem and as a remarkable collectivity of mini-ecosystems and to the seamless interwoven-ness they share between themselves. In a few paragraphs, Buhner is able to span the magical and the scientific, and the specific and the universal, that all support Nature's complexity, intricacy, balance, and clarity of intention. Let me share his observations with you as follows:

> Since their emergence some 500 million years ago, Earth's land plants (99 percent of the biomass of Earth) have acted in an intimate dance with the animals and bacterial decomposers to keep Earth's atmospheric gas ratios and temperature remarkably constant. It is the plants who keep temperature constant and who, as they expanded throughout Earth's landmasses, increased the atmospheric content of oxygen from 1 percent to its current level of 21 percent. Without plants, life as we know it would not exist.
>
> Plants breathe in carbon dioxide (CO_2) molecules and during photosynthesis they break them apart; they keep the carbon atoms and breathe out the oxygen. The percentage of oxygen in the atmosphere rose through the plants keeping carbon atoms in their bodies (sequestering). It is kept high through the burial of carbonized plants (charcoal from fires) and the burial of plants as peat, coal, and oil, Only about 0.1 percent of Earth's plants are permanently contained in this carbon "sink," but it is enough to keep oxygen levels high. The rest of the carbon atoms in plants recycle: Any kind of combustion, whether it is logs burning in a fire, bacteria decomposing decaying plants, our bodies slowly burning the foods we eat, or using oil-derived gasoline to power our cars, releases carbon back to the atmosphere as carbon dioxide once again.
>
> High atmospheric oxygen allows rapid chemical processes to occur; all growth accelerates. Animal muscle, which needs a minimum of 10 percent atmospheric oxygen to function, develops. Decaying matter is processed quickly and rocks experience increased bacterial and environmental weathering, which breaks nutrients free for living organisms. For optimum functioning, the ecosystem has to keep oxygen above 15 percent (the point at which fires will burn and large land animals can easily function) and below 25 percent (to prevent uncontrolled raging fires).

Over time, plants have developed specific leaf shapes and leaf positioning to make this process as efficient as it can be. Leaves alternate around a stem or spread out in a flat fan on branches so that those growing above cast a minimum of shading on the leaves underneath. Maximum photosynthesis-capable surface area is exposed. The upper surface of each leaf processes energy from the sun while the underside engages in gas exchange through tiny opening called stomata.

Stomata are essentially tiny lungs. Surrounding them are muscle tissue (much like the diaphragms in our bodies) that constrict and relax, causing the individual stoma to open and close. Basically, plants breathe just like we do. When an individual stoma is full, the opening closes and carbon dioxide and any other usable molecules are separated from the air. What remains, along with the oxygen generated from the breakdown of carbon dioxide, is released back to the atmosphere as the stoma opens again and breathes out. This cycle is powered by sunlight; at night the plants rest, photosynthesis stops, the stomata are closed. But animal and bacterial respiration and fires do not stop when sunlight is not available; they continue to produce carbon dioxide. Earth's levels of carbon dioxide rise at night and lower during the day — Earth's breathing on a 24-hour cycle. Over a hundred billion tons each of oxygen and carbon dioxide are cycled this way each year.

To keep their airways moist, plants transpire: they take up, or hydraulically lift, water from deep in the ground and breathe it out when they exhale. On a hot summer day, a mature cottonwood tree can breathe out 100 gallons of water an hour. It is so much cooler under a tree or in a forest not so much from the shade cast by trees' leaves, but from the incredible amounts of moisture that the trees are exhaling. Forests breathe out so much water vapor that from space it is actually possible to see the rain forest creating the clouds that precipitate later as rain. Forests help cool Earth by keeping the air moist, by making clouds, by making rain.

Hydraulic lifting goes on 24 hours a day. At night, when their stomata are closed, the trees, and all deep-rooted plants, deposit the water they are bringing up just under [the] surface of the soil. Some they will use for transpiration the next day, but about two-thirds is used by neighboring plants as their water supply. Trees literally water their community. Whenever forests are removed — sometimes only half a forest has to be cut — the air and soil begin to dry up, rain becomes scarce, fires are common, and the land starts to become desert.[1] (Buhner 142-145)

---

[1] [From endnote in Buhner's Chapter Seven:] Jonathan Horton and Stephen Hart, "Hydraulic lift: A potentially important ecosystem process," *TREE* 13, no. 6 (June 1998): 232-35.

*identifying frequencies and
Nature's energetic blessings* | *x*

There are also more esoteric perceptions about the energetic gifts of trees as highlighted by Virginia Essene and Irving Feurst in their co-authorship of <u>Energy Blessings from the Stars</u>. A conversation between them develops as follows:

> **VE:** Can you say more about why our beautiful planet's gridwork is incomplete and has been weakened — to our disadvantage?
>
> **IF:** The gridwork as it now exists is seriously incomplete because necessary frequencies are missing due to a series of interrelated historical calamities. One of these involves the demise of the Celtic Earth Keepers, as previously mentioned. The Celtic Earth Keepers also used chanting and toning to bring in divine, subtle sound frequencies. They knew how to utilize Stonehenge to spread those frequencies throughout the planet's gridwork system. There were also other frequencies missing due to misuses of powers in ancient Egypt, which caused the subsequent withdrawal of certain initiations by the Spiritual Hierarchy. A series of calamities also occurred that preceded Egypt, going back to ancient Lemuria and Atlantis. That's really where the problems with Earth's gridwork started. Subsequent events, from ancient Egypt to modern times, are like knocking over a row of karmic dominoes set up in ancient Lemuria and Atlantis.
>
> **VE:** So these damages to the gridwork affected human consciousness and their ability to use energies appropriately.
>
> **IF:** Absolutely, and the missing frequencies in the Earth's gridwork system affect us all in our daily lives very profoundly in ways that most people don't realize. Many people who are sensitive to energy have the feeling that there's something missing, that their energy body is not quite right, and that this lack goes deeper than the influences of their family of origin and of the society in which they now live. It's very important to understand that although our subtle bodies are made up of subtle matter, it is still matter and it must be renewed and replenished! In our physical body we know that cells divide and that we produce new cells as a result of the food that we eat. In a similar way, the subtle bodies have matter that is subject to the law of entropy and over time degrades and must be replaced. Where does this replenishment come from?
>
> Let's take a look at the subtle mental body as an example. Most of the matter in our mental body is made from energy that we absorb from the Sun. The second most significant source of the matter in our mental body comes from trees, and there's a very profound connection between human mental bodies and the subtle energy field of trees. Many people sense this at an intuitive level. They know that when they are next to a tree their thinking is clearer and they feel more at peace. Because there are frequencies missing from the Earth's gridwork system, there are also very important frequencies missing from the energy field of trees. Consequently, there are necessary frequencies missing from our mental bodies. . . .

VE: In nature, we go to the forest or the mountains, the oceans or the deserts, and we really feel physically invigorated. Sometimes that can be interpreted as a spiritual and an emotional uplift, too. And of course we must honor the physical body's oxygenation process!

IF: . . . And it is . . . [also] true that trees . . . have a profound effect on our emotional bodies. Indeed, there are these very intimate links that exist between the different kingdoms of nature — between the mineral kingdom, the animal kingdom, the plant kingdom, and the human kingdom — which must not be disrupted. People are becoming familiar with the concept of ecology on a physical level, and in a similar way realize you can't disrupt the subtle energy fields of any one kingdom without affecting all kingdoms.

VE: So our feelings that we're not as powerful as we should be, that we can't do all the things that we'd like to do, not only come from what you would call a psychological lack of worth and so on, but from a very deep inner sensory level of dissatisfaction. I hear many people saying how hard it is to be here on the planet knowing that they have something missing that can't quite be identified.

IF: Yes, many people have those feelings, and when they realize that there is some reason for them that can't be ascribed to just their family of origin, their society, or their environment — they often look for other reasons. These explanations might have to do with alien sources interfering with the Earth or something related to the DNA level. But the most important thing to emphasize is that the source of these feelings is not something exotic but is literally right under our feet. It's the very Earth — it's the water we drink and the air that we breathe — which lack certain energy frequencies. Indeed the reason these feelings can be so strong is because this lack surrounds us all the time in our daily life. We can't get away from the fact that everything we do is connected to Mother Earth.

These missing frequencies also influence people's spiritual development. Many people have had the experience of clearing themselves of certain negative thought forms only to have those return very quickly, leaving them at a loss to explain why it is so hard to remain clear of these unwanted thought forms. Of course, there are many reasons for this. However, one explanation is that our mental bodies are simply not as strong as they really should be at this point in time. If these missing frequencies were present in the Earth's gridwork, and therefore in the trees and in our mental bodies, it would be much easier for people to clear negative thought forms out of their mental bodies. Then more often we would all feel the way that we do mentally and emotionally when we're in a forest, in nature.

VE: The Cosmic Consortium and the Sirian coordinators of these seven energy blessing gifts to humanity and to the planet, which this book explains, come to help us achieve a greater sense of balance. . . .

IF: Indeed as the Earth's missing frequencies are filled-in, everyone will find it more joyful to be in a body. This will be particularly true for people who are consciously aware and sensitive to energy. There can be a real tendency for people to desire escaping from the body if they are sensitive to energy and notice the feeling that something is missing. However, the body is here for a reason, and we see that even when people evolve spiritually and become enlightened, they don't disappear in a puff of smoke or a flash of white light. They're still here in a body. *The real purpose of humanity's spiritual evolution is not transcendence but wholeness. We are not here to abandon the body but to unify body and spirit.*

As the missing frequencies get restored to the Earth's gridwork it will become easier for people to enjoy the experience of being in a body. Let us be grateful that many masters are working to help bring about this shift in the Earth's gridwork and have been working at this for centuries. These include the masters of our own Planetary Hierarchy and many non-terrestrial masters. . . . When the World Teacher does appear the whole process of restoring Earth's missing frequencies will be greatly accelerated, for this is one of the functions of the World Teacher. It cannot be over-emphasized that the World Teacher will come to develop a spirituality that links people even more deeply to the Earth and that increases people's appreciation for Mother Earth and their own bodies." (Essene, Energy Blessings 219-222)

---

[11] ". . . [O]ne of the great tragedies in the history of Christianity is the loss of the systematic passing on of the esoteric teachings and energies of Jesus.[12] Fortunately, these teachings and energies have not been completely lost. Fragments do survive in scattered locations of the globe even though they have been lost as a coherent system.

One of the important things to understand about any great spiritual leader is that such a leader always passes on both exoteric, or outer teachings, and esoteric, or inner teachings. Any teacher of any subject who is a good teacher will teach different people in different ways depending on their level of consciousness and willingness.

It's also important to understand that the purpose of the esoteric teachings is not to create some kind of an elite. Esoteric teachings are a natural outgrowth of this universal principle of good teaching as well as several other important facts. One is that some of the most important truths about the universe are difficult to believe when you first hear them, and if they are revealed prematurely, a person is likely to reject a truth that is very important for their development. The second point to understand about esoteric spiritual teachings, which distinguishes them from purely intellectual pursuits, is that advanced spiritual practices can lead to the development of various supernormal powers which a good spiritual teacher does not want to pass on indiscriminately.

Esoteric teachings exist in all great spiritual traditions, and even in the New Testament we see places where Jesus tells things to the disciples that he does not tell to the general public. So part of the tragedy of current Christianity is that in an admirable attempt to be democratic — this attempt coming from the recognition that all of us are equal before God — people have corrupted and disempowered the original Christian teachings by denying their esoteric component. But this need not be a permanent situation because the spiritual forces that are guiding humanity are hoping that the full esoteric teachings that Jesus meant to pass on can be brought back." (Essene, Energy Blessings 218-219)

[12] Related to this thought please see: Barbara With, "Jesus of Nazareth," Party of Twelve: The Afterlife Interviews (La Pointe, Wisconsin: Mad Island Communications, 1999) 141-172.

*inviting possibilities and
partnering with Nature*

By way of rounding out our conscious embrace of the gifts and energy blessings of our trees and plants, I would like to share the uplifting and thought-evocative content of a seminar I've recently attended.[13] Our teacher has been David Crow, author of In Search of the Medicine Buddha and licensed acupuncturist, medical herbalist, loving and empathic aromatherapist and practitioner of other natural healing systems and traditional Asian healing arts.[14] He suggests that there are five primary root issues fueling illness in the United States today. He perceives them as follows:

1. socio-economic stress and its direct impact on the nervous system
2. availability of food and its nutritional quality
3. environmental pollution and its bio-accumulable quality and quantity and the cyclical nature of its water, soil, and air sequence
4. negativity of our own thoughts and thought patterns amplified by a generic lack of trust and by our spiritual emptiness. David emphatically reminds us of the profound link between our thoughts, our sense of spiritual connection or disconnection, and our physical health. And he has interactively pondered with us the implications of our disconnection from nature, a nature he observes as the unfolding of Creation — and the same nature for which many indigenous and a decreasing collectivity of non-industrialized cultures have long held an exquisite reverence. He posits that much of the Western world's stress and depression heralds from the way the spiritual bits and pieces don't fit together. And advancing these positions toward their logical conclusion, it is indeed likely that a sense of oneness and spiritual communion with the natural environment could evoke a reconnection with our spiritual history and a re-sketching of both our spiritual and our exoteric futures.
5. epidemic proportions of iatrogenic illnesses and deaths omnipresent in hospitals and clinics in the United States today.[15-21] David has included here observations on the brilliant healing and supportive role of essential oils with ample emphasis placed on their outstanding ableness to help persons transition from the synthetics and the side effects of pharmaceuticals to a co-blending of what the body already knows how to process and to the nurturing, nutritional, and toxin-evacuative properties of the natural. Indeed allopathic medicine actually extends dis-ease in certain circumstances and regularly increases morbidity with pharmaceuticals in general and with antibiotics in particular.[22-26]

[13] From information presented by David Crow in his seminar "Pharmacy of Flowers," Crestone, Colorado, 29 June 2004.

[14] ". . . [Crow] is the founder of the Center for Sattvic Medicine, which provides holistic therapies derived from his studies with Chinese, Ayruvedic, and Tibetan doctors. He is dedicated to promoting the Dharmic principles and earth-based wisdom of traditional healing arts as a path to ecological restoration and revival of spiritual cultures" (Crow 376).

[15] *Iatrogenic* describes doctor-caused illnesses — mis- or over-prescribed drugs, etc. I would like as well to comment on secondary (as in less direct) implications of iatrogenic disturbances. In our hospital settings today, with many persons with similar and dissimilar issues collected under one roof, the effects of mis- or over-prescribed medicines, misdiagnoses, and malpracticings for whatever reasons, arrive onto the emotional, mental, psychological, spiritual and physical terrain of patients who are already profoundly affected. In many cases these same patients are deeply compromised by the interior and exterior terrains of their own family members and friends, by the interior and exterior terrains of the family members and friends of their fellow patients and by the interrelationships and interrelatings ongoing between staff and staff, staff and doctors, and staff and doctors and patients. This transference of emotions is a very real and impactful substrata consistently overwoven with disturbances of a iatrogenic nature. (Phillips)[16]

[16] Please see *Sources Cited* under Phillips, "Iatrogenic Settings."

[17] "Sensitive healers through the ages have observed that thoughts and feelings are composed of subtle atmospheric energies, infused with etheric gunas.[18] By elevating the patient's shen[19] with compassion, loving kindness, and happiness, a sattvic[20] doctor can increase the therapeutic effects of medicines and treatments. Doctors manifesting rajasic symptoms of stress and unhappiness negatively affect patients, who are already sensitized by pain and suffering. Ayurveda recognizes this phenomenon and encourages physicians to cultivate sattvic mental states in order to benefit their patients. . . .

Sattvic healing philosophy believes that the more deeply we are connected to our inner divinity, the healthier we become; the role of medical treatment is therefore regarded in Ayurveda as secondary to the more important work of supporting a patient's spiritual evolution. . . .

The ancient doctor-sages taught that the practice of medicine is an excellent path for cultivating sattvic virtues, which can lead the physician to moksha, spiritual emancipation. This idea is clearly elucidated in the teachings of the *Tsa Gyu*, which state that by embodying the sattvic qualities of Sange Menla, a physician may reach enlightenment. When physicians integrate meditation and prayer into the everyday work of medical practice, healing becomes a spiritual path; thoughts, actions, and speech are purified with sattvic mindfulness, and the clinic is transformed into a sacred temple. Every interaction with the patient can become an expression of the six paramitas, the boundless disciplines of morality, generosity, concentration, diligence, wisdom, and patience, which lead to transcendent fulfillment. Upon the altar of uncontrived morality, the physician places offerings of selfless generosity. With one-pointed concentration, he performs the ritual of healing with tireless diligence. Guided by the wisdom of mental equipoise, he patiently nurtures the transmutation of sickness into health. Thus, the healing arts become a supreme vehicle for realizing meaningful inner refinement, and a profound sadhana[21] that opens the secret lotus of the heart.

. . . [D]eity reminds us that ultimately, the physician is not the healer: it is the plant kingdom that provides the different elements, qualities, and tastes which balance the body. By approaching the art of healing as a servant of Creation's compassionate intentions, generously sharing sattvic medicines given freely by the earth to benefit our bodies and minds, physicians can find personal satisfaction and professional fulfillment, and avoid suffering for themselves and others.

Herbal medicine, when practiced with conscientious skill and compassionate motivation, transmutes the primitive feeling-consciousness of the plant kingdom, which is ruled predominantly by the tamas guna into a sattvic art and science. Most herbs used in clinical practice are sources of food-grade phytonutrients with minimal toxicity and are therefore unlikely to produce side effects; those that are highly toxic will create problems only if not properly purified and administered. The side effects of most common herbs tend to be mild and transient, and long-term use does not create the insidiously complex levels of iatrogenic complications seen with synthetic pharmaceuticals. The majority of herbs used as medicines possess the sattvic virtues of being nutritive and immune-supporting, regulatory and balancing to physiological disequilibrium, rendering them incapable of curing chronic and degenerative illnesses." (Crow 268-271)

[18] Gunas translate as qualities (Crow 259).

[19] Shen translates as spiritual presence (Crow 375).

[20] Sattvic translates as that which is best for everyone (Crow 363).

[21] Sadhana translates as spiritual discipline (Crow 28).

[22] Let us address morbidity as Henry Lindlahr, M.D., has in his Philosophy of Natural Therapeutics and as Robert Stevens, director of and professor at the New Mexico School of Natural Therapeutics in Albuquerque has in numerous classes 1999-2004 as that that the body cannot digest — spiritually, mentally, emotionally or physically.

[23] "Somewhere in the evolution of the modern mind, we lost our connection with the simple, sensitive intelligence of the heart and our affinity and empathy for the land, its plants, and its creatures. The dissociation from spirit and nature affects all areas of culture, including medicine. Altruistically seeking to alleviate illness, yet desensitized by reductionistic science in pursuit of financial profit, medical research has both battled diseases and inflicted new suffering. In its complex relationships with industry, agriculture, the military, and biological sciences, modern medicine has given birth to valuable creations, but has also spawned inventions and practices that should never have been released into the world. By ignoring the voice of higher intuition, the deeper guidance of conscience, and the feelings of other sentient beings, researchers have perpetrated dangerous, painful, and fatal experiments on people, animals, and the environment. Physicians have taken the Hippocratic vow of ahimsa, nonviolence, yet the institution of allopathic medicine is troubled with a legacy of iatrogenic sickness, political corruption, and toxic wastes, the dark shadows of marigpa[24] that poison the sacred art of healing.

One of the deepest wounds inflicted upon the world by the loss of sattvic wisdom in medicine is the adverse mutation of microbial intelligence caused by modern antibiotics. Antibiotics from botanical sources, such as mushrooms, algae, lichens, and alkaloid-producing plants, have been used throughout history. Undoubtedly, people have perished experimenting with some of these substances, and others have suffered at the hands of incompetent herbalists and physicians. Unlike the mass-produced synthetic drugs of modern allopathy, however, classical Asian medicines have never been a source of widespread iatrogenic sicknesses, a threat to the health of large human and animal populations, or a danger to the food chain and environment. Instead, holistic medical systems such as Ayurveda, and the gentle paradigm of unity their philosophies teach, are emerging as important solutions to the declining effectiveness of antibacterial medications and rising microbial virulence. Traditional indigenous plant-based medicines and therapies, unlike the biologically aggressive compounds created by our nature-dominating society, are nourishing, strengthening, cleansing, and rejuvenating, and promote individual, social, and ecological equilibrium.

The 'germ theory' of allopathy is an excellent example illustrating the differences between the contrasting paradigms of classical Asian and modern medicines, the worldviews they evolved from, and their consequences. Pathogenic bacteria, when they interfere with normal physiological functions, are responsible for many of the most serious diseases of humans, animals, and plants. With the advent of microbiology and the development of the germ theory of pathogenesis, a new world of pharmaceutical possibilities emerged, based on the creation of 'miracle drugs' to kill bacterial invaders.

In the land of Ayurveda, where contagious febrile diseases born of poverty and pollution are an everyday part of life, physicians have also developed medicines which are highly successful for treating bacterial infections, using plants and minerals with antibiotic properties. Yet, surprisingly, Ayurvedic philosophy places relatively little emphasis on the microbial origins of sickness or eradication of bacteria; instead, it promotes immunological development through dietary measures, herbal supplementation, and hygienic daily conduct." (Crow 340-341)

". . . [F]or a disease to flourish, several factors are important. . . . Diseases are not there because the bacteria are there. . . . It is our body's reaction which constitutes a disease" (Dr. Singh, Crow 342).

"We live on a planet that belongs to bacteria. They are the most abundant organisms on earth, whose collective weight is greater than all other forms of life combined. The human body is inhabited by highly intelligent microbial communities composed of hundreds of types of bacteria, viruses, yeasts, and other organisms, in unimaginable numbers. On one square inch of intestine there are more microbes than humans on the planet. A trillion bacteria live on our skin, 10 billion reside in our mouth, and 100 billion are flushed down the toilet after every bowel movement. Over 300 different types of bacteria swim in the digestive tract. Overall, about 100 trillion individual organisms consider each of our bodies as their home. Almost all of them live in a harmonious synergistic existence with the others, and with us.

These organisms play an important role in sustaining our health. The microbes of the digestive tract help

attaching themselves to the intestinal wall and competing for nutrients, they form a protective colony against invading organisms. They produce natural antibiotic substances, stimulate the production of antibodies to fight infection, and destroy pathogenic organisms. We owe our health, digestive capacity, and immunity to the complex intelligence of the microbial communities within us." (Crow 342-343)

"Louis Pasteur was the father of microbiology and the originator of modern science's germ theory. His ideas about germs being the causative agents of disease were widely debated by scientists of his day. At the end of his life, Pasteur expressed his final views, which were the same as Ayurveda's. 'The microbe is nothing,' he declared, 'the terrain everything.'

Although the Ayurvedic pharmacopoeia contains numerous botanical drugs with highly effective antibiotic properties, developing the body's resistance by restoring equilibrium within the terrain of tissues and humors is the primary goal of treatment, while subduing microbial toxins is secondary; most formulations for infectious febrile conditions simultaneously 'attack' pathogens and 'support' vitality. The emerging pharmaceutical industry in the West, however, found the pursuit of a 'magic bullet' that could simply eradicate germs far more lucrative than preventive measures such as lifestyle modifications and enhancement of immunity using natural methods. Four antibiotic generations later the long-term consequences of this 'attacking' philosophy are now appearing in the microbial kingdom." (Crow 343-344)

"Under the influence of antibiotics, the weakest strains of bacteria die off and the hardiest mutate to survive. These increasingly virulent strains pass on new genetic information to their offspring, and more powerful substances are required to control each succeeding generation. Common types of bacteria have mutated into a wide variety of new forms, appearing in outbreaks of 'superinfections' and medically resistant forms of old diseases such as tuberculosis and gonorrhea. While strengthening unwanted organisms, antibiotics also weaken the beneficial ones by eradicating the healthy microbial communities of the body. The combined results are decreased immunity and vitality, susceptibility to overgrowth and reinfection by invasive microbes, and accumulation of disease-promoting toxic residues. Using Chinese medical terminology, these effects can be described as 'treating the stem while weakening the root.' This symptomatic approach does not address causative factors. . . .

If scientists had deliberately set out to radically alter the global microbial environment, they could not have found a better way to do so. In the space of a few decades, we have planted the seeds of virulent disorder in the microbial soil; now those seeds are coming to fruition, bringing the end of the antibiotic era. The fundamental shortsightedness of the allopathic paradigm — overlooking and underestimating the far-reaching repercussions of biochemical interference with nature's complex intelligence — is more apparent now than ever. The painful lesson to be learned from medically created diseases is that therapies which compromise human ecology must at least be supported, if not replaced whenever possible, by treatments which strengthen resistance. As modern drugs lose their effectiveness, the spiritual wisdom of the physician-sages and their vitalistic methods of healing will once again play a central role in medical practice. A holistic paradigm emphasizing harmony and compatibility with other forms of life will deepen in the psyche of the world, accompanied by a renaissance of traditional plant-based healing systems such as Ayurveda." (Crow 344-345)

". . . The premature use of antibiotics in the treatment of 'unripened' fevers, . . . causes toxins to migrate through the body, where they become the source of recurring illnesses and, eventually, more serious diseases. . . .

. . . [W]hen an 'unripe' fever is prematurely suppressed, it is transformed into a 'hiding fever.' When colds and flus are mistreated with strong medicines, they can become unresolved conditions that hide in the interior of the body. The illness may appear outwardly cured, but due to its hidden nature it is actually difficult to heal. The analogy used to describe hiding fevers is a fire that has died down, leaving a tiny ember glowing under the cold ashes. This ember contains the dormant toxins of the unresolved fever, which gradually consume the body's vitality and leave it susceptible to reinfection. Secondary factors, such as poor diet or insufficient sleep, function like wind blowing on the ember, which can reignite into a recurrence of the previous illness." (Crow 348)

"The proper management of the early stages of febrile diseases, according to the wisdom of traditional physicians, is to first 'ripen' the fever; this brings the fever to a state of maturity by allowing the body to activate its thermogenic defenses. Following this stage, a fever is then 'consolidated,' meaning the toxins are brought together so they become centered in one location in the body. When this has been accomplished, the final stage is referred to as 'killing' the fever, when medications to subdue and neutralize the toxins are administered. The successful treatment of fevers in this system is based on careful observation of subtle changes within the pulse, tongue, urine, and symptoms, and continual modification of medications. It is a way of practicing medicine that is more personal and time-consuming than is possible in modern clinics.

'One who follows the above three stages can be considered a good physician,' Amchi-la told me. By following this protocol, the immune system is strengthened and developed, the pathogens destroyed, and the phlegmatic 'soil' in which they are thriving restored to health. The result is that children's fevers are completed in childhood, and not perpetuated into adulthood as unresolved allergic syndromes, immune deficiencies, and conditions of chronic fatigue." (Crow 349)

[24] Marigpa translates as spiritual ignorance (Crow 373).

[25] "The limitations of modern medical advances, the weaknesses of allopathy's symptomatic methods, and the dangers of utilizing powerful drugs without a strong scientific and moral foundation are starkly evident. . . .

Even under the best medical conditions, synthetic pharmaceuticals have an inherent flaw which renders them incapable of curing the diseases of the future: they can neither cleanse toxins from the body nor regenerate vitality. Ultimately, all sickness is related to these two physiological processes, which are now under increasing stress from environmental pollution and degradation of the food chain. Without agents to remove the rising accumulation of chemical, metallic, and radioactive poisons in our bodies, especially the liver, and without compounds to enhance and strengthen resistance and immunity, allopathic medicines will become increasingly ineffective and inappropriate. Doctors everywhere are already seeing the human face of the spreading ecological crisis, as more patients come with complex allergic and immunological disorders caused by the multitude of poisonous substances pervasive in our homes, workplaces, and diets. Many physicians are unaware of the origin and scope of these problems, lack the training and methods to treat them, and further complicate the underlying causes by prescribing drugs that add to the body's toxic burden.

Now more than ever, we need the healing gifts given freely by the plant kingdom, to protect and strengthen, nourish and revitalize, cleanse and detoxify, both our bodies and the environment. Plants not only are the medicines which can cure the toxicity syndromes and nutritional deficiencies of the future; they also have the power to purify the earth's elements and remove the environmental causes of future epidemics. When the era of antibiotics has ended and synthetic medicines have failed, the wondrous creators of photosynthesis can heal us with the sunlight, blood-purifying chlorophyll, antibacterial essential oils and alkaloids, vitamins, and complex trace elements stored in their bodies. They also provide, on a global scale, what technology and science cannot: drinkable water, breathable air, and fertile soil.

As the earth sickens and increasing numbers of people are afflicted with illnesses unresponsive to modern drugs, the demand for botanical medicines will increase, and skilled practitioners of natural therapies will continue gaining respect and recognition. Herbal products are already a rapidly growing multibillion-dollar global industry and one of the fastest-developing fields of agriculture. But classical Asian medicines and their holistic philosophies are not merely medical and economic trends; more important, they are helping countless people find healthier, more satisfying lifestyles, and raising collective awareness of our dependency on the well-being of the environment. The growing need for herbal medicines and traditional healing knowledge could bring about a revolutionary change in social priorities and become a catalyst for the preservation of wilderness, development of nonpolluting plant-based economies, and establishment of sustainable ecosystems. 'Of all the new frontiers of agriculture,' says a World Bank report, 'the cultivation of medicinal plants is among the most powerful for doing good in the world.'

Plants are sustenance for all creatures and when conjoined with human intelligence and compassion, are the basis of civilization. A global horticultural renaissance, motivated by deteriorating collective health, economically stimulated by lucrative botanical markets, and guided by the holistic philosophies elucidated by Ayurveda and other traditions, could transform destructive ignorance into life-sustaining wisdom, and bring about the blossoming of an earth-centered spiritual culture." (Crow 330-332)

[26] "Perhaps the most valuable contribution Ayurveda has to offer the world is its definition of health: equilibrium among the humors, tissues, transformations, and wastes; and happiness of mind, senses and soul. True health is the result of living harmoniously with the forces of nature, and the fruit of a culture's flowering spiritual maturity. Long-term ecological equilibrium, the global foundation of individual health, can be brought about only through sattvic consciousness guiding a society that loves, respects, and nurtures human, plant, and animal life." (Crow 352)

David neither posits nor imagines that natural medicine per se is the solution — favouring rather a coordinated introduction of urban forests, ecovillages, herbal sanctuaries, and community gardens from which could evolve our dream *of* and Mother Nature's intention *for* free pharmacies for all — community by community.

When people become involved in the creationing and sustaining of such eco-endeavours, then all five primary root issues are addressed. David further points out that the cultivation of medicinal plants addresses issues extending critically beyond a nucleus of health and health care. Indeed he sees four global benefits ensuing:

As # *1* he sees non-toxic, plant-based, sustainable healthcare which at some future point could translate into free medicine for everyone in the manner of a "people's pharmacy." (He sees causes of disease clustering predominantly and generically around issues of excess and deficiency.)

As # *2* he sees herb projects being made economically sustainable, as with the example of the extraordinarily financially lucrative and spiritually and physically benefitting qualities of the floral oils. (Consider that the going price of one ounce of agarwood oil in Nepal is a thousand dollars — and that in the distillation of every gallon of rose essence, a hundred gallons of rose hydrosol are produced. Consider also that whole economies are being developed around pockets of ecotourism introduced with the cultivation of lavender and rose. And consider finally the possibility of herb projects becoming economically sustainable: observe the Nepalese farmers who have been taught by a sattvic benefactor to terrace and to farm their hillsides with roses for which they now receive a large sum — and these, the same farmers who formerly were receiving only a few rubles for their potato crops.)

As # *3* he sees that the cultivation of medicinal herbal crops for the extraction of their essential oils, could and would massively contribute to the protection of the environment. Nature and humanity-benefitting agricultural techniques could be taught and practiced, techniques that would be both soil rejuvenating and sustaining.[27] Consider for example the following possibilities for naturally protecting our soils:
- Letting grasses such as palmerosa and jamrosa suck up the floodwaters of the yearly monsoons in Nepal and in this way giving to farmers some control over the flooding.

- Planting vetiver to help hold the top soil. It prevents soil erosion by percolating the rainwater back into the ground, recharging this ground water and performing what we might call phytoremediation. Additionally, vetiver plants deal unusually with pesticides — sucking them up and breaking them down — and subsequently "eating" them.

(Let us note with proactive concern that historically one of the main reasons for the demise of civilizations has been the extreme disregard of its peoples for the caretaking of their precious soils.)

And finally, as # *4* he sees the addressing of the spiritual through the preservation and restoration of our natural culture and heritage — encouraging the plants, the trees, and Mother Nature to come back into balance. Indeed we so need to have them and an awareness of their relationship with our planet in our everyday lives and experiencings and daily in our consciousness.

Several other observations could be collected to emphasize the parameterlessness — indeed the illimitable quality and quantity of Mother Nature's gifts. We can cite example after example. Is it well-known that the banyon tree (of Biblical fame) gives the most oxygen to our planet of any single plant or tree? Or that frankincense and myrrh trees are the mainstays of desert ecology and participate in entire networks of symbiotic relationships which are destroyed if one kills or majorly disturbs them by harvesting them unnecessarily? Is it taught to us or even randomly known or emphasized that in our proximity with trees in forest settings and elsewhere, we are blessing ourselves and our immune systems with the immune system of trees? Trees

---

[27]Several additional examples could be of interest here:

1. We could cite a two hundred square mile area in Bulgaria known as the Valley of the Rose — where the Damascena rose is cultivated. She is intercropped with the white Alba rose and apparently the Red rose strengthens the white immunologically and vice versa.

2. We could cite as well that since the source of sandalwood oil is the heartwood of the tree and since the whole tree has to be cut down to harvest her great gift, replanting on a regular schedule in the old growth forest when trees are cut is urgent. Knowing that a really superb quality of oil is obtainable only after forty years (though some may consider thirty years an acceptable timeframe) is also key if one is involved with the propagation of this majestic being. That quality oils come from sandalwood trees grown in old growth forests rather than on plantations is another salient tidbit one had best observe. Indeed sandalwood trees need to be grown with other trees exactly because they use the roots of these other trees for their nourishment.

3. And finally as a third example, we could cite the way in which patchouli and agarwood are successfully intercropped. Patchouli can be harvested three times a year while waiting the twenty-odd years for the agarwood to begin to bear fruit. In this way the farmer already receiving an income from the patchouli on a regular basis can afford both to cultivate the agarwood and to wait the appropriate forty to eighty years for her optimal maturity.

produce the atmosphere and the oils are their immunity in a way of speaking. So when we breathe the atmosphere they create, we're breathing their immunity, which then strengthens our own. I find it enchanting to note that the exquisite fragrance of the Damascena rose is secreted maximally on the morning of the full moon and that every flower emits an orb of aromatic molecules and emits this orb in accordance with a biorhythm. These molecules respond to cosmic events as in the case of the full moon cited above. Different flowers appear to have differently sized orbs — for example the dawn blooming jasmine has a ten foot aura while the champa flower appears to have an aura five times that of the jasmine.[28]

There is a deep biological interrelatedness of All — a deep and sacred relationship between the atmosphere and our breath — a deep and profound relationship between consciousness and matter.[29] There is a biological unity between us all and we can bless our planet with the harmonious mental states of our gratitude exactly for this unity and this community. Let us offer forth a prayer of joyful appreciation for our plants and for our trees and for the gifts of their most sacred essences and let us extend our gratitude to all who have shared and do continue to share in this ballet of our ongoing evolution and re-awakening.

---

[28] Crow, "Pharmacy."
[29] Ibid.

part the third:

appendices

an annotated anthology

sketching a dream of fluidity and trust
revelations of life unveiling
beyond limitation and fear

In light of the extraordinary range of understandings currently blessing our planet, I have wanted to assemble this admittedly extensive collection of appendices to introduce in the caring words and phrases of their authors those concepts of nature, frequency, healing, earth history and galactic geography that can help us, as conscious and inwardly caring residents of this blessed planet, make sense of the phenomenal gifts of Ages Shifting concurrent with the closing of a five thousand years long Mayan calendar. I am aware that the length and range of this collection of appendices could seem overbearing or maybe just awkward and I would therefore ask with extreme humility that they be received and seen in a slightly tenderer light. If they seem too lengthy or broad ranging as they attempt to paint a backdrop for medicinal aromatherapy's future on our planet, perhaps you could more easily scan or sum them up as an extended collection of one or two word topics in preference to omitting them altogether since to me these informations have seemed so relevant as to be needfully posited in order to examine aromatherapy's future without fear or negativity.

My intention here is to honour both myself and my readers with increased awareness so that fear elements alluded to earlier can be emotionally shifted into frameworks of desire, intuition, grace, and compassion and all increasingly filtered through a diaphanous veil of joyous anticipation. Just imagine if as a result of such efforts, fear were gently rested and as gently transformed into loving gratitude and a child's most innocent enthusiasm? Curiously the fears just referenced are repeatedly and unintentionally invoked by trance channels and others ultra familiar with metaphysical axioms and New Age language and beautifully able to describe the possibilities of consciousness's awakening. These fears are especially drawn forth by the facile use of a language and of terms and concepts too little familiar to those listening or overhearing and beg for reverent care in our use of a metaphysical and spiritually productive idiom.

So often we are either less inclined to insist or perhaps just not knowing that there exists neither a checkerboarded terrain of rights and wrongs nor the linearity of a Candylanded map — only Allness, Unity and a Communion that welcomes all choices and does not see them on a hierarchical continuum or on a continuum of polarities. They are seen rather with a sixth dimensional logic and as a blending of experiences from both extremes so that balance can be embraced through the knowing of both. In further considering the role of medicinal aromatherapy into the future, it seems meaningful to visit a few of the scenarios scattered across the tapestry of pasts, presents, and futures that support visions of potentiality and the revelation of all that

sketching a dream

is and all that is exquisite *about* the medicinal grace and wisdom of Mother Nature as offered us in aromatherapy.

With this in mind, I would like to sketch in a thumbnail-sparse style with various allusions to such facets of the continuum of our esoteric history as the Galactic Federation, the Mayan prophecies etc. Concurrently, if I can delineate one of alternative healthcare's pivotal theories, I could than better honour the medicinal aromatherapeutic gifts of Mother Nature in our cosmic unfolding and in our more and more rapidly unveiling futures, specific and collective. The theory I would propose to expand is the one linking health and disease with the nutritional continuity of the mental and emotional life styles and the personal tables of contents we each embrace in this incarnation and from preceding ones and from those way into the future from which some of us may have returned.

Clearly to honour the intention of collecting such perceptions would require at least a first volume and quiet likely a second and a third. And for this reason I then prefer to include such nuggets in appendices of extended quotations and in a syllabus of suggested texts sectioned into topics for consideration that are both supporting and extending premises pointed out or alluded to above.

In support of extensive quoting and allusions to topics by quotation, let me emphasize that the exploration of aromatherapy's role in our future is a topic of enormous breadth. Massive amounts of hugely pertinent information exist to honour it and I wish to give every credit to any and all sources I've drawn from, be they books and articles or erstwhile classes and seminars. I should like to include as well the titles of books and the appendixed information referenced above,[30] so that my dancing with this topic ultimately creates a meaningful reference tool both for myself in future research and mentoring — and for others in similar capacities.

---

[30] With my most sincere gratitude to the various publishers as listed on page *vii* who have so graciously accorded us the privilege to include explanatory and descriptive text from volumes for which they hold the publishing rights.

Appendix A: Excerpts from *The Lost Language of Plants*[1]

Certainly my intention in the extended texts of these appendices is not only to bring attention to the informations given but as well to so encourage and so entice those for whom certain areas hold exceptional interest that they may subsequently choose to read or further scan the given text as they begin their enchanted journey, aligning themselves and their intentions in co-creative service with their spiritual families, their chosen planet, and their current and evolving roles in the magics of that galactic life unveiling for each of us.

In this first appendix, I would like to sketch the expansive understandings of Stephen Buhner. Reading his brilliant text on The Lost Language of Plants, we are introduced to stories and examples and the richest diversity of quotations from both sides of the *universal* equation — namely the universe as machine and the universe as sacred intelligence. Indeed we are introduced to both the disaster and the gift of the scientific paradigm with such readable fairness and citings of research that the scientific technocrat with even the smallest shred of integrity is bound to read along and notice facts that he might be either unfamiliar with or if sketchily aware of in the past, not then willing to accord heartfelt attention. Now, however, attention will surely be incurred by this incredible collection of facts and known processes assembled by Buhner. He shares ample facts about the already well advanced and still evolving disaster of our natural environment and blesses us beautifully with a new awareness of Mother Earth's exquisite emotional wisdom and her innate knowingness around balance. For the sake of cataloguing some of these considerations, I'd like to include both quotations and a running index of chapter segments that seem cardinally meaningful so that once again others can use this volume both as a reference tool and as an introduction to areas rarely so well addressed in our schools and universities and subsequently in our social and charitable organizations — collectivities which map the usual progression of social interaction and information gathering for

---

[1] Please see *Sources Cited* under Buhner.

those non-crystalline and non-psychic sectors in a highly individualized and highly mechanistic society (e.g. sectors not yet seamlessly heralding from sixth dimensional realities).

[the role of epistemologies][2]

Nearly all scientists insist that indigenous peoples learned the uses of plants through a lengthy trial-and-error process. There is an immediate problem with this assertion, of course; they were not there to observe it. Their assertion is an assumption, a guess, though so widely repeated it has taken on the mantle of fact (33).

Indigenous peoples were clear, however, about where their knowledge of plant medicines originated. In the vast preponderance of cases, when they were asked, they insisted that their knowledge of plants came, not from trial and error, but from the plants themselves, from visions or dreams or from sacred beings. That their description of the sources of plant knowledge should be so uniform is in itself… amazing. The assumption by scientists that all nonindustrial peoples generated these descriptions out of superstition and ignorance is astonishingly shortsighted and, frankly, not very good science. What is especially striking is that the medicinal uses for plants that nonindustrial people were taught during these experiences correspond nearly perfectly to the medicinal actions of the plants that have been identified through science. (35-36)

… Unfortunately, scientific epistemology has historically made it impossible for most scientists to "see" what indigenous peoples were saying. But what if nonindustrial cultures were not engaging in superstition but describing an actual event? This would mean that there is another way to gather information about the Universe and our place in it than what we call "science." (It may be helpful here to remember that the realization of the double helix structure of DNA came to its discoverer not through scientific study but in a dreamlike state, whole and complete.)

Embedded within the underlying epistemologies of the vast majority of non-industrial cultures are the components of this other way of gathering information. While containing numerous variations, themes, and differences these nonindustrial epistemologies do contain a basic framework that is very similar in a number of areas. Most assert that:

- *At the center of all things is spirit. In other words, there is a central underlying unifying force in the Universe that is sacred.*

- *All matter is made from this substance. In other words, the sacred manifests itself in physical form.*

- *Because all matter is made from the sacred, all things possess a soul, a sacred intelligence or **logos**.*

- *Because human beings are generated out of this same substance it is possible for human beings to communicate with the soul or intelligence in plants and all other matter and for those intelligences to communicate with human beings.*

---

[2] All words within brackets are my words as distinct from those of the author of the given text from which the *Appendix* material has been selected.

- *Human beings emerged later on Earth and are the offspring of the plants. Because we are their offspring, their children, plants will help us whenever we are in need if we ask them.*

- *Human beings were ignorant when they arrived here and the powers of Earth and the various intelligences in all things began to teach them how to be human. This is still true. It is not possible for new generations to become human without this communication or teaching from the natural world.*

- *Parts of Earth can manifest more or less sacredness, just like human beings. A human being can never know when some part of Earth might begin expressing deep levels of sacredness or begin talking to him. Therefore it is important to cultivate attentiveness of mind.*

- *Human beings are only one of the many life-forms of Earth, neither more nor less important than the others. Failure to remember this can be catastrophic for individuals, nations, and peoples. The other life in the Universe can and will become vengeful if treated with disrespect by human beings.*

This outline, in a very rough way, represents, perhaps, the oldest epistemology of humankind and was present in most historical cultures on Earth. Cultures codified this in differing ways, described it in different words, rigidified it as religion in varying forms. But beyond its varying forms of expression in different cultures and beyond its classification as religion it represents a way of describing human relationship with the Universe and Earth. If all the emotional connotations are removed, this epistemology is not so different from some of the descriptions that scientists have of the world, the Universe, and human beings. (For example: $E=MC^2$; green plants gave rise to the oxygen atmosphere that allowed the evolution, the birth, of human beings; by studying the Universe we can gain knowledge and not be ignorant of the things around us; failure to live in an ecologically balanced way can and probably will lead to environmental disaster.) There are, as well, a number of major differences. Though historical indigenous and nonindustrial peoples were exceptionally gifted empirical observers, they did not believe that the Universe is a great machine which, by disassembly, examination, theoretical exploration, analysis, and study can be understood, its workings made plain. They ascribed to the Universe livingness, interior depth, intelligence, soul, and a central unifying spirit at its core. (37-39)

> Burrowing creatures, such as prairie dogs, open millions upon millions of tubes in the soils of Earth.... [Bill] Mollison [in *Permaculture*] notes, these "burrows of spiders, gophers, and worms are to the soul what the alveoli of our lungs are to our body." As the moon passes overhead the underground aquifers rise and fall and Earth breathes out moisture-laden air. This exhalation of negative-ion-charged air through the many fissures and tubes opened by the burrowing creatures helps create rain.
>
> How could indigenous peoples have known this? By all our standards of scientific knowledge they could not. We have neglected to realize that indigenous peoples have always had access to the finest probe ever conceived, one that makes scientific instruments coarse in comparison, one that all human beings in all places and times have had access to: the focused power of human consciousness. (61)

What is interesting to me is what happens to human behavior, individually and culturally, when differing epistemologies are taken on and internalized. The more widely that science is internalized by cultures and individuals, the more clearly they are significantly affected by such internalization. This leads to questions: Does the wide acceptance of the epistemology of science, specifically seeing universe-as-machine, support successful habitation of Earth? Does it support healthy habitation inside a human life for individual human beings? Does it maintain the health of cultures?

Science is really a remarkable human invention. But in all the excitement of its usefulness the fact that it *is* an invention is often forgotten. As with all human inventions it possesses limitations, unexamined assumptions, and design flaws.

Because of the strong conflicts between fundamentalist Scientists and fundamentalist Christians, it is very difficult to examine the limits of science or standard evolutionary theory without being labeled a fundamentalist Christian or unscientific, or even as someone who hates science itself. That there are a diversity of perspectives about science among many different kinds of people is often overlooked. Many scientists and the general public are often unwilling — indeed, will antagonistically refuse — to openly explore problems in the structure of science and their possible ramifications. This unwillingness by so many scientists to self-examine their profession is exceedingly disturbing.

Perhaps science should be more like knives: understood to be a useful tool that, if misused, can be dangerous. Knives can accidentally wound, or even, in the hands of the deranged, be used to kill. Yet individuals and cultures understand the potential danger of knives and allow for it in their daily use. Knives, unlike guns, are not assumed to be inherently evil in contemporary debates nor, like science, to be always beneficial and harmless.

How science may cut us as a species if we let our attention wander or if a madman gains control of it is not well understood in our culture, and any examination of this aspect of science is often strongly discouraged. This prevents science from being as well integrated into human cultural life as a knife — a useful tool whose strengths and weaknesses are well understood. Because science is assumed to be essentially beneficial with no shadow side it is impossible to know how to use it safely — by cultures or individuals. (45-46)

The internal effects on people of the scientific epistemology are more subtle but just as painful as the effects on the rest of nature. Once the Universe becomes a machine, no longer alive, once human beings are defined as the only intelligent life-form, a unique kind of isolation enters human lives, a kind of loneliness that is unprecedented in the history of human habitation of Earth. It is a source of many of the emotional pathologies people struggle with. In addition, people begin to judge themselves internally, to identify their level of value according to how much or how well they think. Any internal expressions, perceptions, or thoughts that come from older epistemologies — that are based primarily on feeling or intuition or aliveness in the Universe — they label unscientific, irrational, unreasoning or illogical. Such thoughts and perceptions, it is assumed, have less value, are based on improper assumptions about the nature of reality, and are therefore something to be discounted, dismissed, degraded. This dynamic has become so ingrained that people routinely monitor and censor perceptions that are contrary to universe-as-machine. And so people cut themselves off from the Universe in which they live; they become passengers on a ball of semi molten rock hurtling through the Universe. They internally denigrate and deny their most basic experiences of the livingness of the world in which they live, their connection to it, and the importance of that connection. The interior wound.

The tension between these two perspectives — Universe as alive and universe-as-machine — is readily perceivable. (51)

[Let us consider one further adjunct of the scientific epistemology — poetically phrased in a passage from Louis Pascal's famous Ninth Working Paper of December, 1991[3]:]

> Reality is a seamless whole where virtually everything affects virtually everything else. There are, however, various concentrations of interaction of causation, and we have somewhat artificially divided these up into "disciplines." There is a certain amount of overlapping at the edges of many closely related disciplines, and this is good. There is a certain amount of bridging that is done even between more distantly related disciplines, and this is also good. But there is much about the structure of reality that is missed by this artificial classification. There are important connections between information fitted into separate disciplines that are being badly overlooked. These weaken our man-made structure. And there are important gaps in the seams between adjacent disciplines. We have a leaky structure where information that we need to encompass is leaking out.... And these inherent weaknesses in our way of dealing with reality by dividing it into self-contained, graspable chunks, become magnified by social interactions within each discipline that tend to draw it into itself and thereby widen the gaps: the tendency of disciplines to develop a jargon and often a dogma and to some extent a clique, all of which make it more difficult to bridge the gaps. This is further magnified by a tendency for research not to push out the borders of a discipline at the edges, nor to establish connections to other disciplines, but rather to superspecialize and plunge even deeper into the minutiae of the subject until it is impossible to be an expert except by spending all one's effort in the field, with little or nothing left over to become even cursorily familiar with other disciplines.
>
> – Louis Pascal, "What Happens When Science Goes Bad" (182)

the loss of biophilia and biognosis

One of the first movements toward bonding with the Earth is when we learn to crawl....

Our eyes move over the landscape; it is filled with interesting colors. Our ears listen; Earth is rich with sounds. We begin to put things in our mouth, tasting the Earth, sticks, and grass. We smell the scents in which we swim, the smell of plants, and dogs and cats. Our hands feel the landscape that we travel across. We feel the emotions that these things generate. All of this finds a place inside us; we store it away. Biophilia begins to awaken.

As children age the process extends itself. The four-year-old may spend a lot of time playing alone in the yard, sitting beneath a tree, or talking to flowers. By eight years of age the first period of lengthy time in nature without adult supervi-

---

[3] Louis Pascal, "What happens when science goes bad: The corruption of science and the origin of AIDS: A study in spontaneous generation," University of Wollongong, Science and Technical Analysis Research Programme, Working Paper No. 9, December 1991.

sion has occurred. Perhaps it is an hour spent catching minnows in a creek, or a morning chasing frogs, or a day collecting interesting feathers and rocks. The necessity for unsupervised time in wild landscapes is important during this later time. The accumulating years of exploratory contact and experience of nature coalesce into biophilia, into a deep bonding with Earth. The regular contact with nature, growing longer and more unsupervised as time goes by, allows the genetic predisposition for biophilia to awaken.

The continual immersion in nature where the bonding process is supported and encouraged allows it to deepen into **biognosis** — direct, depth knowledge of nature that cannot be reduced to the assembly of a collection of bits of accumulated information. Knowledge of the complex interactions of natural systems or the contribution of individual members is gained without being able to pinpoint each step in the process. There may in fact be no steps; it comes in dreams or a flash of understanding. The knowledge, because of immersion in biophilia, is directly communicated from the landscape, plants, or animals themselves. There may be a predicating factor that bursts the knowledge into awareness, but the many elements that went before are and remain unconscious — an expression of the ancient interplay between organisms interwoven in the matrix that gave them birth as species — an interplay between species that are, at their core, relations.

Unfortunately, biophilia and biognosis are being interrupted throughout the world, especially in Western cultures. The loss of biophilia leads directly to the loss of biophilia-dependent biognosis and this creates large scale risks for us as a species. Certain holistic aspects of the workings of Earth and its ecosystems cannot be understood without utilizing the natural and ancient human capacity for biognosis — the grasping of gestalts of whole-system functioning.... Without an activated capacity for empathy with other living things we risk becoming ever more disruptive of the ecosystem functioning of the planet.

... Biophilia should normally awaken in children as they grow, then continue to develop in complexity throughout the rest of their lives. Without specific initiating factors (regular early contact with an experientially living Earth, for one), biophilia does not awaken in its proper time and biognosis never develops.

(Still, it **can** awaken in later life; it is a fundamental need. Biophilia can awaken at times of intense stress or change, especially at major life shifts when prior developmental stages are being recycled, such as the movement into puberty, middle, or old age. But all too often the factors that interfered with its original emergence derail these later expressions as well.)

There are a number of factors that I think are at the root of why so few people are developing a deep bonding with the living Earth — factors contributing to the loss of biophilia. Arguably among the most powerful are: the epistemological perspective that the Universe (and Earth) is not alive but simply a machine assembled from a large number of parts; the loss of natural regular access for children to nearby wild places that contain a diversity of life-forms; public schooling; and television. (60-63)

... Human beings over the course of their evolution have had frequent contact with a wide variety of wild animal and plant species and ecosystem structures. These were and are intricately bound up in what and how human beings are. Such contact generates specific types of responses in people **that have been a part of human experience since our species began.** As the number of wild animals, plants, and healthy ecosystems are depleted — as local ecosystems become homogenized — children have less and less occasion to come into contact with them.... There is then no activating factor to generate biophilia. Though children often do have contact with domesticated pets, house plants, and the lawns surrounding their houses, this is not the same thing. If you have ever had the opportunity to look into a wolf's or coyote's eyes, even in a zoo, it is immediately apparent that they are significantly different in nature from dogs.

A two-thousand-year-old tree or an ecosystem filled with a tumultuous, complex riot of interacting plant species **feels** markedly different from a lone sapling surrounded by the grass planted in the front yard of a new housing development, or the Norfolk pine in the corner of the kitchen. The green orderly lawns surrounding children's homes do not bear any relationship to the up-and-down, uneven landscapes filled with giant, craggy outcroppings of the immeasurable ancient stones of Earth that wild landscapes often possess.

Although often difficult for reductionists to accept, differing landscapes each project different and distinct **feeling tones**....

By not having close contact with natural ecosystems that evoke the feeling tones and meanings with which human beings have evolved, occasional, regular encounters with the wild intelligence of animals inside their own world, and regular experience of wild, untamed plants growing as they have for millions of years, something is not awakened in human beings. It is then impossible for us to understand that animals sometimes climb to the top of hills simply to look at the stars, or that when a wild herd animal is killed the rest of the herd will sometimes pause and wait until, like a sigh, the spirit of the slain animal passes.

As the loss of species and habitats spreads farther and farther it is less and less likely that children will encounter wild ecosystems with a diversity of life during the period of their development when biophilia normally awakens. Those ecosystems they do encounter are more and more likely to be unhealthy. Few people have explored what the likely result will be of children regularly encountering only diminished and unhealthy landscapes. Will any biophilia at all be generated in diminished landscapes? What kind of biophilia will it be? Will or can it be healthy? (65-67)

... [About television, Buhner suggests that it] is often derided ... in general, for the wrong reasons. Television is of pervasive importance because it is used to fulfill a basic need that we all have: it is intricately bound up with our need to dream. Dreaming is a basic need like food, clothing, shelter, or touch....

Dreaming is necessary because human beings have an innate need to make sense of things, to understand who and what they are, to continually process and interweave the **meanings** they encounter each day into the fabric of their lives.... The purpose of dreaming is to allow the unconscious mind to work with the meanings of one's life, both interior and exterior. By this process a person integrates meaning into the fabric of his character, his life takes on more and more meaning as time goes by, he deepens — becomes less shallow, more alive and real.

Most dreaming is never consciously remembered, but during all of it the unconscious works with the material offered up to it through daily living to extract meaning, to understand our place and relationship to the world, the Universe, and life. It is an organic process as integral to human health and life as food, this need to work with **meaning** through dreaming. And like all our other basic needs, it has been taken by human beings and, over time, developed into art. Before printing, dreaming was crafted as art through storytelling, eventually developing more complexity as theater. After printing, storytelling followed a new tack and developed as art through written fiction. They all involve our human capacity and need to dream.

In listening to storytelling or reading fiction, as we listen, we enter a dreaming state — a fictional dream as the writer John Gardner named it.... We enter a dream world, we forget ourselves, our conscious mind sleeps.

Each of us has had the experience of suddenly being awakened from such a fictional dream — by the insistent ringing of the telephone or a sharp knock at the door. It startles us awake as if from a deep sleep and it takes a few minutes for us to recall ourselves, for our conscious mind to begin functioning again. Yet even as we answer the phone or the door, the meanings, experiences, or people we were dreaming about linger in the mind like a taste on the tongue or the fading chords of music in the ear.

The more accomplished that storytellers and authors become, the more their stories' structures resemble the organic process of dreaming and the more deeply we enter their fictional dreams. Fiction and storytelling become *great* when, in addition, the meanings embedded within them are the deep and important meanings that we grapple with daily in out lives and nightly in the deepest core of our dreaming....

People have the capacity to grasp deep meaning in stories from the subtlest of cues....

These kinds of embedded meanings build up in works of fiction as they do in dreams....

Over time, storytelling branched off into written fiction, and theater branched into moving pictures. With "movies" storytelling even more closely began to resemble dreaming because dreaming contains such sounds and images. Eventually this branching dynamic produced television, but television possesses a number of significant differences compared to movies. With television, dreaming is no longer an irregular, isolated event like sleep-dreaming, the theater, or a trip to the movies (events set off in time and space as important), but a habit casually undertaken at any time one wishes. It has been flattened as well. Television's stories contain meanings that have been processed to be broad and shallow rather than specific and deep in order for them to apply to the largest number of people. And the dreaming process is continually interrupted by commercials — a unique shift in our evolutionary history of dreaming.

Dreams are by their nature individually generated and their meanings apply specifically to the person dreaming.... Because the dreams that storytellers embody in books usually only apply to a few people or are poorly done, the vast majority of novels rarely sell more than a few thousand copies. A novelist such as Tolkien or Hemingway, whose work moves many millions of people, is uncommon. (There is, of course, a difference between books filled with the kind of meaning that occurs in dreams and books that are essentially lengthy gossip. Gossip fills an entirely different need than that filled by dreaming. Books that are only compelling story line are, in many respects, just another form of gossip.

Television is to dreaming what junk food is to real food.... Dreaming, like food, is a basic human need and was once present in only limited amounts....

Television is not a special event, set aside in time, like the theater, books or movies. It runs twenty-four hours a day, seven days a week. There are very few people in the Western world who do not have a television set at all. Television needs a lot of programming and by nature and function those programs must affect the most people possible. This can be done by consistently *producing great fiction — an impossibility, there are only so many Tolkiens or Hemingways — or else by lowering the depth of the dream. Making shallow dreams that can affect the broadest number of people. Television.*

As a result, people are continually exposed to dreaming that works with very shallow and homogenized meanings reflective of one particular industry and way of thinking. The deep unconscious responds to the material as it does to anything that resembles dreaming — it works with what it gets, deriving what meaning it can. Because the level of meaning is so shallow people begin to live more and more in a world with less and less access to deep meaning. More and more life is lived in front of a television dreaming dreams that have been generated only to be palatable to the most millions. Less and less does dreaming come from life itself. Children begin to take these dreams and the meanings derived from them and interweave them into the fabric of their characters. It is no wonder that teenagers feel that life is meaning-less....

A further disruptive aspect of television is that the dreaming that people receive, unlike all other dreaming, is not continuous; it is interrupted by commercials — specific dreams designed to get the viewer to purchase goods and services. Commercials interrupt the process of dreaming — they awaken the dreamer every ten to fifteen minutes. This is much like letting someone go into REM sleep and then waking them up every six minutes or like sitting down to a good book and having to answer the phone six times an hour. With television it happens not once but always. This corrupts a process the unconscious expects to be continuous.

The majority of dreams on television are derived from a human-centered, universe-as-machine perspective, and as such they are also an expression of our cultural mythology of a dead universe. The only life and meaning that exist are assumed to be in human communities. And those meanings in television that are developed as representative meanings of human communities occur along a very narrow and limited range of exploration.

But regular encounter with the wild was once normal and is essential to healthy dreaming. We are historically made to need such dreaming. The homogenized shallow dreaming of television, by its nature, does not meet that basic need.

Our culture no longer recognizes that each aspect of the wild, natural world possesses its own meaning and feeling tone, a **numen***. These, encountered at random in different sequence and frequency by each human being as they mature, accumulate in number by the day, week, month and year. They are incorporated, in an unpredictable manner, in the unconscious dreaming of each person during sleep. The unconscious weaves them into the meaning that makes up the fabric of each individual human being. Without this experience of diversity of life that has always been an integral part of human life we cannot become whole... . Stephen Kellert says, "The degradation of this human dependence on nature brings the increased likelihood of a deprived and diminished existence — again, not just materially, but also in a wide variety of affective, cognitive, and evaluative respects. The biophilia notion, therefore, powerfully asserts that much of the human search for a fulfilling existence is intimately dependent upon our relationship to nature."*$_{17}$[4] *(68-75)*

---

[4] The numerals for all author generated footnotes will be subscripted and can be found at the conclusion of each *Appendix*.

Sacred Choices

an arbitrary beginning

Since their emergence some 500 million years ago, Earth's land plants (99 percent of the biomass of the Earth) have acted in an intimate dance with the animals and bacterial decomposers to keep Earth's atmospheric gas ratios and temperatures remarkably constant. It is the plants who keep temperature constant and who, as they expanded throughout Earth's landmasses, increased the atmospheric content of oxygen from 1 percent to its current level of 21 percent. Without plants, life as we know it would not exist. . . .

High atmospheric oxygen allows rapid chemical processes to occur; all growth accelerates. Animal muscle, which needs a minimum of 10 percent atmospheric oxygen to function, develops. Decaying matter is processed quickly and rocks experience increased bacterial and environmental weathering, which breaks nutrients free for living organisms. For optimum functioning, the ecosystem has to keep oxygen above 15 percent (the point at which fires will burn and large land animals can easily function) and below 25 percent (to prevent uncontrolled raging fires).

Over time, plants have developed specific leaf shapes and leaf positioning to make this process as efficient as it can be. Leaves alternate around a stem or spread out in a flat fan on branches so that those growing above cast a minimum of shading on the leaves underneath. Maximum photosynthesis-capable surface area is exposed. The upper surface of each leaf processes energy from the sun while the underside engages in gas exchange through tiny openings called stomata.

Stomata are essentially tiny lungs. Surrounding them are muscle tissue (much like the diaphragms in our bodies) that constrict and relax, causing the individual stoma to open and close. Basically, plants breathe just like we do. When an individual stoma is full, the opening closes and carbon dioxide and any other usable molecules are separated from the air. What remains, along with the oxygen generated from the breakdown of carbon dioxide, is released back to the atmosphere as the stoma opens again and breathes out. This cycle is powered by sunlight; at night the plants rest, photosynthesis stops, the stomata are closed. But animal and bacterial respiration and fires do not stop when sunlight is not available; they continue to produce carbon dioxide. Earth's levels of carbon dioxide rise at night and lower during the day — Earth's breathing on a 24-hour cycle. Over a hundred billion tons each of oxygen and carbon dioxide are cycled this way each year.

To keep their airways moist, plants transpire; they take up, or hydraulically lift, water from deep in the ground and breathe it out when they exhale. On a hot summer day, a mature cottonwood tree can breathe out 100 gallons of water an hour. It is so much cooler under a tree or in a forest not so much from the shade cast by the trees' leaves, but from the incredible amounts of moisture that trees are exhaling. Forests breathe out so much water vapor that from space it is actually possible to see the rain forest creating the clouds that precipitate later as rain. Forests help cool Earth by keeping the air moist, by making clouds, by making rain.

Hydraulic lifting goes on 24 hours a day. At night, when their stomata are closed, the trees, and all deep-rooted plants, deposit the water they are bringing up just under the surface of the soil. Some they will use for transpiration the next day but about two-thirds is used by neighboring plants as their primary water supply. Trees literally water their community. Whenever forests are removed — sometimes only half a forest has to be cut — the air and soil begin to dry up, rain becomes scarce, fires are more common, and the land starts to become desert.[1] (142-145)

the plant as seed

Plants put into their seeds the unique chemistries necessary for them to grow when they are released into the world. They also put a large number of compounds in the seeds themselves or on their seedcoat (certain tannins, alkaloids, lactones, phenolic compounds, and flavonoids) to protect them from soil microorganisms. As a result, some seeds can remain viable in soil for years or decades until they sense the right conditions for germination.[4] These chemical mechanisms can be quite sophisticated. *Datura stramonium* (also known as jimson weed), for example, coats its seeds with hyoscyamine and scopolamine. These two alkaloids protect the seed from microorganisms and also prevent its germination. When rainfall sufficient for germination leaches the compounds from the seed coat, the seed begins to sprout. The alkaloids disperse through the soil, where they are still strong enough to inhibit other plants and microorganisms in the immediate vicinity.[6] Parent plants often vary the amounts and types of chemicals they deposit in their seeds so that each seed will process slightly different compounds in slightly differing quantities, helping ensure its survival.[7]

Though dormant, seeds are constantly analyzing the makeup of their external environment through the same complex feedback loops that all plants use. At the moment they sense that just the right conditions exist for them to germinate, seeds begin to release unique combinations of plant compounds such as abscisic and gibberellic acid, cytokinins, and ethylene, which regulate germination and are bioactive at extremely low concentrations — less than 10 ppt.[8] Each seed also contains enough sugar (in the form of starch) to fuel its growth until it can begin photosynthesis on its own. At germination the seed releases an enzyme that begins converting the stored starch to sugar. Each plant uses information from tightly coupled feedback loops between itself and the environment to determine the composition and release of all these chemistries.

A newly developing plant embryo, unlike a human embryo, has no sterile womb in which to grow and so, in a sense, makes its own. As soon as germination begins, the new plant starts releasing compounds through its tiny root system to essentially make a sterile zone around the emerging rootlet. This action protects the seed from harmful organisms and makes space in the soil for its growth. *Solidago altissima* (a species of goldenrod) and *Erigeron annus* (white-top fleabane), for example, release combinations of six to ten different matricaria and lachnophyllum esters (ME and LE) to reduce the growth of plants nearby and so make room for themselves in the soil. Like many phytochemicals these particular esters are highly active at very low concentrations. Dehydromatricaria ester (a type of ME) and LE cause a 50 percent growth inhibition in nearby plants at only 10 to 20 parts per million (ppm).[9] These compounds have a half-life of one to two days before they biodegrade and must be regenerated through photosynthesis. Still, they are present long enough and in enough concentration that young seedlings can generate a "zone of protection" around themselves until they sprout. All new seedlings have their own unique types of compounds to help them grow. Their environmental feedback loops tell them what chemicals to release, in what combination, and in what quantity.[10]

Because of the diversity of life a new seedling can encounter, its seed chemistry must be able to affect a wide range of fungal, microbial, and plant metabolisms and structures: stomatal function, cell walls, membranes, mitochondria, chloroplasts, chlorophyll production, nuclei, nucleoli, cell division, photosynthesis, respiration, protein synthesis, lipid (or fat) synthesis, enzyme formation, mycorrhizal binding, nodulating bacteria, mineral uptake, and water uptake, among others.[11] The chemicals that are generated can be quite elegant and specific in their actions. For instance, certain seed-released phenolic acids and flavonoids depolarize the electrical potential difference across cell membranes while at the same time altering the permeability of the membranes, thus affecting mineral uptake by the cells of the roots, and, as a result, the growth of the plant.[12] Juglone, created by walnut trees and their seedlings, can completely inhibit respiration and photosynthesis in nearby plants and microorganisms.[13] And normally non-water-diffusable lipids can be combined with other compounds to diffuse them through soil, affecting plant germination and growth.[14] *Zapoteca formosa*, a plant that grows in northern Brazil, for example, emits a complex mixture of compounds at germination: nonprotein amino acids, djenkolic acid, taurine, 1,2,4,6-tetrathiepane, dimethyl-disulfide, 2,4-dithiopentane, benzothiazole, and a large number of unidentified sulfides and non sulfur compounds. The root exudate is so strong that a single germinating seed in a petri dish will completely inhibit the germination of 50 lettuce seeds, 25 tomato seeds, or 25 *Acacia farnesiana* seeds. None of the compounds show any inhibitory activity alone, but when combined in exactly these ratios they produce one of the strongest germination inhibitors known.[15] Whatever the mode of action used by the plant the result is the same: space in the soil for the new seedling to sprout. (146-149)

plant aerosols

Plant chemistries also move into the ecosystem and soil through their release as aerosols from the surface of plant leaves and, sometimes, stems. Chemical volatiles that are released to guide or call pollinators make up some of this flow, but plants also release huge quantities of terpenes and other aromatics as well. The world's evergreen forests release more than 1,000 megatons (two trillion pounds) of terpenes per year.[82] Additional trillions of pounds of terpenes are released by such plants as yarrows, artemisias, and ambrosias, and these all combine with trillions of pounds of scores of other aromatic volatiles. They infuse the atmosphere, sometimes traveling great distances, and fall as a constant rain down onto the soil, plants, and microorganisms beneath the plants that generate them. Plant communities live in clouds of unseen aromatic volatiles. They breathe them in; their bodies are coated with them. These volatiles are significantly bioactive in plant systems; plants can be anesthetized by gases such a chloroform, just like people. Some of the volatile terpenes that are released, cineole and dipentene for instance, are potent inhibitors of oxygen uptake by mitochondria. This inhibits respiration by bacteria and newly germinating seedlings but does not appreciably affect mature plants. Other volatiles, such as the coumarin esculin and a number of sesquiterpenoid lactones (arbusculin-A, achillin, and viscidulin-C), significantly increase the respiration and stomatal activity of mature plants.[84] (In certain ecosystems the terpenes released by such plants as creosote bush, eucalyptus, certain artemisias and salvias, are so inhibitory that few other plants can grow under their overstory.)[85] Just a few of the actions of plant terpenes: They purify the air, modulate plant emergence, enhance the respiration of the plant community, feed into mycelial networks, and play an essential role in the formation of humic acid.

Plants, and their chemistries, do even more, of course. They are intimately interwoven into the lives of all organisms on Earth. And the roles of plants are still more complex. They exist not for themselves alone; they create and maintain the community of life on Earth, they produce the chemistries all life needs to live, and they heal other living organisms that are ill. (169-170)

elder, nurse and community plants

... In many ecosystems the density of plant species growing between the archipelagos is much greater than in the Sonoran and they blend imperceptibly into one another. A hundred acres of meadow might have three primary bush types scattered irregularly within it and fifty to one hundred subordinate plant species in different densities associated with each of them. Even in a forest each tree has scores of plants associated with it. They each form archipelagos; the tree archipelagos in forests are just very close together. Tightly coupled feedback loops exist between all archipelagos in an ecosystem. The intercommunication between them shapes and maintains their ecosystem and its responses to stressers. How ecosystems respond to environmental stressers changes completely with which keystone species are at the centers of their archipelagos.[12]

The formation of archipelagos — the movement of keystone species in ecosystems such as the Sonoran — often takes place over a 400- to 500-year period and is initiated by episodic ecosystem events that are unknown and are not predictable. They are initiated by environmental feedback cues whose nature is unrecognized and unsuspected by the majority of researchers.[13] Quite often, before it can establish itself in a new location, a keystone species must have a plant that goes first and prepares the way. These initial species, usually selected from among the community of plants that grow with keystone plants, are the outriders, the plants whose emergence signals the movement of plant species in mass, and the slow shifting of ecosystems in response to Gaian feedback loops. These plants move first and essentially determine what keystone plants will grow where and when. In a way, they act as "filters" through which keystone species are sifted.[14] This is often done by plants such as the Artemisias and Ambrosias who, when the soil is ready, send out chemical cues telling the keystone species where and when to send its seed. Though wind, ants, and burrowing animals may sometimes disperse keystone seeds to the new locations, researchers have found that mere wind and animal dispersal patterns explain how the seeds move. The distances are too far, the dispersal patterns too unusual.[15] But by whatever means, the seeds answer the chemical call sent by the nurse plants.

In the Great Basin of Utah and Nevada, sagebrush, and Artemisia, established the community that pinon pine needs. It nurses the pinon until it is old enough to grow on its own: changing soil chemistry, providing unique chemistries for the emerging seedling, protecting it from the vagaries of life.[16] And in the Mojave Desert approximately three-quarters of young creosote bushes are found under Ambrosia shrubs.

Paloverde trees also germinate in areas first inhabited by Ambrosia species. The Ambrosia acts as a nurse plant, raising the paloverde seedling until it is large enough to live on its own. And though the endangered saguaro cactus will establish itself under ironwood it more often prefers paloverde. Thus the saguaro depends on the Ambrosia that comes, unseen by modern eyes, sometimes centuries before.

> ... The name literally means "not mortal" and is named after the food of the gods that, when eaten, confers immortality. *Ambrosia* species are givers of life. (Commonly, Americans call them "ragweeds.") (180-182)

the dangerous loss of plant diversity

The diversity of plant species has been labeled by most scientists as redundant, and unnecessary; the plants themselves have been labeled resources placed here for the use of Man, insentient, and weeds. These care-less attitudes engendered in people by universe-as-machine epistemology have resulted in tremendous reductions in plant diversity throughout the world — in natural systems, medicine, and agriculture. Such loss of plant complexity interrupts healthy ecologies (internal and external) and allows the emergence of disease everywhere it occurs. The Monarch butterflies that sequester toxic cardiac glycosides in their bodies as larvae, for example, are experiencing serious depredation from birds during overwintering in Mexico. Many of the more toxic milkweeds that the larvae once fed on have decreased in abundance while other, less toxic milkweeds have increased, due to changes in human land use and agriculture. Because the butterfly larvae are feeding on less-toxic plants they build up fewer defensive chemicals in their bodies and birds can eat them with impunity. This is affecting the intricate butterfly/larvae/milkweed relationship and subsequently the health of the ecosystems in which they occur.[69]

The internal ecology of living organisms also needs continual inputs from wild plant chemistries to remain healthy. Large herbivores, for example, whose rumens contain more than 100 different types of symbiotic bacteria and uncounted numbers of protozoa and fungi, regularly seek out and eat multiple plant combinations depending on their level of health and particular bodily needs. The ingested plants' secondary compounds alter the composition of the communities in the rumen, input different chemistries, and shift levels of health.[70]

But these kinds of internal ecologies are altered significantly if wild plant chemistries are diminished in the diet through such things as monocropped food plants. Such plants contain considerably fewer secondary compounds than wild plants. In consequence, living organisms that eat them as a steady diet are deprived of the normal complex chemistries that their species evolved with over, sometimes, millions of years. For example, pigeons, when fed a diet that in people causes goiter, will develop polyneuritis — an inflammation in multiple nerve pathways. When the pigeons are allowed to return to their normal ecosystem diet the disease disappears. The birds always harbor the microbes that generate the condition, but the chemical diversity of the plants and insects normally eaten by pigeons does not allow the disease to occur.[71] The internal ecology of animals is maintained by plant chemistries just as soil rhizospheres are.

In people, increases in cancers exactly parallel the decrease of diverse plants as foods and medicines. In 1900, for instance, more than a hundred different types of apples, fifty different types of vegetables, and thirty different types of meat were commonly found in markets depending on the season. Many were wild harvested and their chemistries were much more highly diverse and potent than the foods we buy now. Many of those wild-gathered plants contained the multiple types of cytotoxic, antimutagenic, and cell-division inhibitory compounds regularly ingested in human diets prior to 1900. The iKung bushmen of the Kalahari Desert, as an example, regularly eat more than seventy-five different plants in their diet in one of the harshest ecosystems on Earth; cancer is virtually unknown. (They additionally work less hours than we do, have a high caloric intake by American standards, and spend most of their time in what we call "leisure pursuits.")

Historically, human beings have eaten between 10,000 and 80,000 different food plants in their diets. Some they intentionally grew, most they wild harvested. The combination of plants shifted from season to season, with local plant populations, and in response to the needs of the people. The kinds of diseases we see now are virtually unknown with such diets. Complex plant combinations keep disease conditions in check in people, just as they do in pigeons and in ecosystems.$_{72}$ (205-207)

Plants are, in essence, ecological medicines. They do not require expensive factories to make them, they do not discharge pollutants into the environment, they have far fewer side effects (internally and externally), they are renewable, and the knowledge of their use is not held in the hands of a few experts but, like plants in ecosystems, is diffused throughout the cultures that use them. They are also very inexpensive. . . . And of course, in communities that work with wild plant medicines, who pick and prepare them themselves, they cost nothing at all (209).

Scientists who embraced universe-as-machine labeled indigenous and folk understandings of plant medicines useless superstition and set about removing them from the sum total of human knowledge. The pressure of Western medicine on herbalism, on folk and indigenous healing, has initiated the destruction of systems of biognosis-generated healing hundreds of thousands of years old. It is not so different than the destruction of older forms of agriculture and their replacement with modern agribusiness farming technologies. Universe-as-machine has not created a disease-free life in a Garden of Eden filled with bountiful food, but rather has initiated the increasing loss of plant species throughout the world, loss of knowledge of their use, waste that will not go away, diseases more virulent and pervasive than any known before, and ecosystems in disarray. (209)

plants and people

Plant chemistries, unlike pharmaceuticals, are released into the world for a reason. Each chemistry a word imbued with import, all together a language that possesses its own grammar and syntax. Its own underlying epistemology. Scientists study the vowels and consonants and how they are put together to form plant words, but they do not study their meaning, nor the intelligence or intent that gives rise to that **meaning.** Too often they insist there is no meaning, for, as anyone can see, plants have no brain. Still, each complex assemblage of expressed plant chemistries is a sentence of communication, carrying specific messages, imbued with meaning. And the world receives those meanings and responds.

Plant communications are like stones in water. The ripples they create move throughout ecosystems; they wash up against us. That we take plant words in through our nose or our skin or our eyes or our tongue instead of our ears does not make their language less subtle, or sophisticated, or less filled with meaning. As the soul of a human being can never be understood from its chemistry or grammar, so cannot plant purpose, intelligence or soul. Plants are much more than the sum of their parts. And they have been talking to us a long time. . . .

*The plants release Earth's subtle chemistries through their intertwined, interdependent synaptic feedback loops faster and more complexly than researchers, or anyone, can write them down. Their meanings pile one on top of another until the linear mind is overwhelmed. They shift the fabric of our world, touch us with meanings, in ways too complex for our conscious mind to grasp. Nevertheless, we can grasp them. They come in gestalts to the attentive mind and caring heart, concise reflections of plant and Earth interrelationships, in knowledge whole and complete: "The trees are the teachers of the law." It is not necessary to have a degree in English to understand the meaning of words. Training in chemistry is irrelevant to understanding the meaning conveyed by plants. A four-year-old does not worry about it; she sits under a tree talking with flowers. For thousands of generations, human beings in all cultures on Earth have known that plants (and **all** of nature) express meaning and that there is intent behind it. They have been listening to and accumulating those meanings; they have been building a biognosis-generated oral library of knowledge of the world and humanity's place within it. (225-227)*

*The plants have long been our teachers and healers.... **We are their** children; they are not our property. As with all children, when we hurt, the nature of their relationship to us leads them to want to help us. When the ancient Greeks named certain plants **Ambrosias** — givers of life — this is something they understood.*

The ancient Greek and Roman, folk and indigenous plant names and plant usages that developed over millennia came out of this perspective. The use of plants as medicines connects us as people to those ancient traditions, to the environment of which we are a part and from which we came, to the meanings that the plants generate; for a million years human beings have been healed by them. Wendell Berry has captured the knowledge of this succinctly:

> *Herbalism is based on relationship — relationship between plant and human, plant and planet, human and planet. Using herbs in the healing process means taking part in an ecological cycle. This offers us the opportunity consciously to be present in the living, vital world of which we are part; to invite wholeness and our world into our lives through awareness of the remedies being used. The herbs can link us into the broader context of planetary wholeness, so that whilst they are doing their physiological/medical job, we can do ours and build an awareness of the links and mutual relationships.*[4] *(228-229)*

Appendix A

author endnotes

chapter 4

17 Steven, Kellert, "The biologcal basis for human values of nature," in *Biophilia Hypothesis*, ed. Edward O. Wilson and Stephen Kellert (Washington D.C.: Island Press, 1993), 42-43.

chapter 7

1 Jonathan Horton and Stephen Hart, "Hydraulic lift: A potentially important ecosystem process," *TREE* 13, No. 6 (June 1998): 232-35.

5 Alan Putnam and Chung-shih Tang, "Allelopathy," in *The Science of Allelopathy*, ed. Allan Putnman and Chung-shih Tang (New York: Wiley and Sons, 1986).

6 John Lovett, "Allelopathy: The Australian experience," in ibid.

7 May Berenbaum, "The chemistry of defense," in *Chemical Ecology*, ed. Thomas Eisner and Jerrold Meinwald (Washington, DC: National Academy of Sciences, 1995).

8 Putnam and Tang, "Allelopathy," in *The Science of Allelopathy*.

9 Kenneth Stevens, "Polyacetylenes as allelochemicals," in ibid., 219-20.

10 Nicholaus Fischer and Leovigildo Quanijano, "Allelopathic agents from common weeds," in *The Chemistry of Allelopathy: Biochemical Interactions Among Plants*, ed. Alonzo Thompson (Washington, DC: American Chemical Society, 1985).

11 R. E. Hoagland and R. D. Williams, "The influence of secondary plant compound on the associations of soil microorganisms and plant roots," in ibid., F. A. Einhellig, M. Stille Muth, and M. K. Schon, "Effects of allelochemicals on plant-water relationships," in ibid., Paul Keddy and Luachlan Fraser, "On the diversity of land plants," in *Ecoscience* 6, no. 3 (1999): 366-80.

12 Nelson Blake, "Effects of allelochemicals on mineral uptake and associated physiological processes," in *The Chemistry of Allelopathy*.

13 G. P. Waller and F. A. Einhellig, "Overview of allelopathy in agriculture, forestry and ecology," in *Biodiversity and Allelopathy*, ed. Chang-Hung Chou, George Waller, and Charlie Reinhardt (Taipei, Taiwan: Academia Sinica, 1999).

14 Fischer and Quanijano, "Allelopathic agents from common weeds."

15 John Romeo, "Functional multiplicity among non-protein amino acids in Mimosoid legumes: A case against redundancy," in *Ecoscience* 5, no. 3 (1998): 287-94.

82 James Lovelock, *Healing Gaia* (New York: Harmony Books, 1991).

84 Einhellig, "Mechanisms and modes of actions of allelochemicals," in *The Science of Allelopathy*.

85 Nikolaus Fisher, "Mono and sesquiterpenes as plant regulators," in ibid.

chapter 8

12 Shahid Naeen, et al., "Plant neighborhood diversity and production," in *Ecoscience* 3, no. 3 (1999): 355-65; J.P. Grime, "Benefits of plant diversity to ecosystems: Intermediate filter and founder effects," in *Journal of Ecology* 86 (1998): 902-10.

13 Steve Archer, "Tree-grass dynamics in a *Prosopis*-thornscrub savanna parkland: Reconstructing the past and predicting the future," in Ecoscience , No. 1 (1995): 83-99.

14 Grime, "Benefits of plant diversity to ecosystems."

15 K. D. Bennett, "The power of movement in plants," in *TREE* 13, No. 9 (September 1998): 339.

16 Ragan Callaway, "Positive interactions among plants," in *The Botanical Review* 61, No. 4 (October 12, 1995).

69 J. B. Harborne, *Introduction to Ecological Biochemistry* (London: Academic Press, 1982) 94.

70 A. Chesson, "Plant degradation by ruminents: Parallels with litter decomposition in soils," in *Driven by Nature*, ed. G. Cadisch and K. E. Giller (Wallingford, England: CAB International, 1997).

71 Peter Tompkins, and Christopher Bird. *The Secret Life of Plants* (New York: Harper and Row, 1973) 225.

72 Timothy Johns and Laurie Chapman, "Phytochemicals ingested in traditional diets and medicines as modulators of energy metabolism," in *Phytochemistry of Medicinal Plants*, ed. John Amason, et al. (New York: Plenum Press, 1995).

chapter 10

4 Wendell Berry, quoted in *HerbalGram* 26 (1992): 50.

Appendix B: Excerpts from In Search of the Medicine Buddha[1]

In considering both the economics and the health crises in many third world nations, we can readily imagine the gift that cultivating lucrative medicinal crops could be, and would also be in many non-third world nations. We appear to be at such an ecological crossroads today with very real and impactful consequences honouring either choice. We hear such a lot about the devastation of our agribusiness farming and foresting practices and equally and as validly much about the separative consciousness that so often nuances humanity's embrace of the natural environment. There is also a wondrous and surprisingly practical other side championed by David Crow both in his writings and seminars as well as in his urban garden and community pharmacy projects. Earlier in chapter *xi* I have highlighted some of these perceptions that he has so wisely and with such love and firmness of vision, taken from the marriage of his Chinese, Ayurvedic, aromatherapeutic and herbal trainings and from his years of service and of study with his teachers in Nepal. And now here I would like to share with you salient, teaching, and hugely forward-considering passages from his book, In Search of the Medicine Buddha:

> *No one knows with certainty the full range of endangered and recently extinct forms of life, or how their functions are entwined, for we have only begun to glimpse the immense web of complex interrelationships among the microbial worlds, animal kingdoms, plants, and the behavior of the planet's elemental systems....*
>
> *Nor does anyone know what impact the loss of this many plants will have on the microbes, insects, and animals they symbiotically sustain, and in turn, how humanity will be affected. Modern research is finally revealing what indigenous people have taught their children for millennia: our lives depend on the small and seemingly insignificant forms of life we ignore, take for granted, and mindlessly annihilate. With the disappearance of butterflies, birds, and other tiny treasures, plants*

---

[1] Please see *Sources Cited* under Crow.

will be unable to pollinate and reproduce, and the earth's crucial life-support systems may no longer function sufficiently to support humans. The breakdown of wastes will become slower, oxygen regeneration will diminish, soil fertility will weaken, and atmospheric balance will be disrupted. (329)

The limitations of modern medical advances, the weaknesses of allopathy's symptomatic methods, and the dangers of utilizing powerful drugs without a strong scientific and moral foundation are starkly evident....

Even under the best medical conditions, synthetic pharmaceuticals have an inherent flaw which renders them incapable of curing the diseases of the future: they can neither cleanse toxins from the body nor regenerate vitality. Ultimately, all sickness is related to these two physiological processes, which are now under increasing stress from environmental pollution and degradation of the food chain. Without agents to remove the rising accumulation of chemical, metallic, and radioactive poisons in our bodies, especially the liver, and without compounds to enhance and strengthen resistance and immunity, allopathic medicines will become increasingly ineffective and inappropriate. Doctors everywhere are already seeing the human face of the spreading ecological crisis, as more patients come with complex allergic and immunological disorders caused by the multitude of poisonous substances pervasive in our homes, workplaces, and diets. Many physicians are unaware of the origin and scope of these problems, lack the training and methods to treat them, and further complicate the underlying causes by prescribing drugs that add to the body's toxic burden.

Now, more than ever, we need the healing gifts given freely by the plant kingdom, to protect and strengthen, nourish and revitalize, cleanse and detoxify, both our bodies and the environment. Plants not only are the medicines which can cure the toxicity syndromes and nutritional deficiencies of the future; they also have the power to purify the earth's elements and remove the environmental causes of future epidemics. When the era of antibiotics has ended and synthetic medicines have failed, the wondrous creators of photosynthesis can heal us with the sunlight, blood-purifying chlorophyll, antibacterial essential oils and alkaloids, vitamins and complex trace elements stored in their bodies. They also provide, on a global scale, what technology and science cannot: drinkable water, breathable air, and fertile soil.

As the earth sickens and increasing numbers of people are afflicted with illnesses unresponsive to modern drugs, the demand for botanical medicines will increase, and skilled practitioners of natural therapies will continue gaining respect and recognition. Herbal products are already a rapidly growing multibillion-dollar global industry and one of the fastest developing fields of agriculture. But classical Asian medicines and their holistic philosophies are not merely medical and economic trends; more important, they are helping countless people find healthier, more satisfying lifestyles, and raising collective awareness of our dependency on the wellbeing of the environment. The growing need for herbal medicines and traditional healing knowledge could bring about a revolutionary change in social priorities and become a catalyst for the preservation of wilderness, development of nonpolluting plant-based economics, and establishment of sustainable ecosystems. "Of all the new frontiers of agriculture," says a World Bank report, "the cultivation of medicinal plants is among the most powerful for doing good in the world."

Appendix B

Plants are sustenance for all creatures and, when conjoined with human intelligence and compassion, are the basis of civilization. A global horticultural renaissance, motivated by deteriorating collective health, economically stimulated by lucrative botanical markets, and guided by the holistic philosophies elucidated by Ayurveda and other traditions, could transform destructive ignorance into life-sustaining wisdom, and bring about the blossoming of an earth-centered spiritual culture. This is the symbolic meaning of Bhaisajyaguru's kingdom of Sudarshan: enlightened consciousness governing a sacred society, which lives harmoniously within a flourishing and healthy natural environment.

Is it possible to create an ecological paradise that nurtures humanity's highest potentials? If this utopian dream cannot be achieved, can nations enjoy prosperity and good health by building their economies on the peaceful and meaningful use of nontoxic renewable resources? If this idealistic goal cannot be reached, can enough people find sustainable livelihoods that will at least ensure a livable world for coming generations? Each of these scenarios is founded on our relationship with the plant kingdom.

If we were to ask the Medicine Buddha, "What can you offer to us to protect and restore the earth?" we need only look to the deity's hand and heart. The mandalic geometry of Sudarshan converges at Bhaisajyaguru's heart, proclaiming that for civilization to thrive, it must be governed by love and wisdom. The deity's hand reaches toward us in the mudra of supreme generosity, showing us the antidote to the greed that has impoverished the world and endangered our children's future. Graceful lapis fingers hold a fruiting myrobalan branch, symbol of the botanical realm's restorative fecundity — upon which rests the success of all human endeavors — reminding us that the earth provides freely, asking nothing to sustain her fertility but gentle care given in gratitude.

When Buddha taught the art and science of healing, the world became a medicinal realm, luxuriously endowed with an abundance of trees, shrubs, bushes, grasses, vines, tiny herbs, and creatures large and small. Sudarshan is not only a mythical kingdom where divine physicians carry on their noble sattvic labors, alchemically pouring elixirs to remove the suffering of beings. Beautiful to Behold is also the answer to the environmental crisis threatening the future of humanity; it is the forest-garden of a spiritual civilization, waiting to be replanted, cultivated, harvested and shared by all. Here, in this green mandala, is a vision not only of past splendor, but of hope for a renewed world. (330-333)

What Dharmic sacrifices will we make to bring the world back into balance? Will we give up our addictions to the fossil fuels and petrochemicals burning the atmosphere, the nuclear plants waiting to explode from old age and sabotage, the tons of carcinogenic pesticides sprayed on the soil, the toxic-spewing industries flooding the world with unnecessary consumer products? Will corporations abandon their ambitions to invent ever more dangerous technologies? Who will renounce the thirst for political power over others? What nation will lay down its weapons to feed its poor? . . . [H]ave [we] chosen to sacrifice the earth and her inhabitants upon the altar of fear and greed[?] (336-337)

. . . Day after day I would listen to the stories of patients seeking help for their deteriorating health. . . .

Somewhere in the evolution of the modern mind, we lost our connection with the simple, sensitive intelligence of the heart and our affinity and empathy for the land, its plants and its creatures. This dissociation from spirit and nature affects all areas of culture, including medicine. Altruistically seeking to alleviate illness, yet desensitized by reductionist science in pursuit of financial profit, medical research has both battled diseases and inflicted new suffering. In its complex relationships with industry, agriculture, the military, and biological sciences, modern medicine has given birth to valuable creations, but has also spawned inventions and practices that should never have been released into the world. By ignoring the voice of higher intuition, the deeper guidance of conscience, and the feelings of other sentient beings, researchers have perpetrated dangerous, painful, and fatal experiments on people, animals, and the environment. Physicians have taken the Hippocratic vow of ahimsa, nonviolence, yet the institution of allopathic medicine is troubled with a legacy of iatrogenic sickness, political corruption, and toxic wastes, the dark shadows of marigpa[2] that poison the sacred art of healing.

One of the deepest wounds inflicted upon the world by the loss of sattvic wisdom in medicine is the adverse mutation of microbial intelligence caused by modern antibiotics. Antibiotics from botanical sources, such as mushrooms, algae, lichens, and alkaloid-producing plants, have been used throughout history. Undoubtedly, people have perished experimenting with some of these substances, and others have suffered at the hands of incompetent herbalists and physicians. Unlike the mass-produced synthetic drugs of modern allopathy, however, classical Asian medicines have never been a source of widespread iatrogenic sicknesses, a threat to the health of large human and animal populations, or a danger to the food chain and environment. Instead, holistic medicine systems such as Ayurveda, and the gentle paradigm of unity their philosophies teach, are emerging as important solutions to the declining effectiveness of antibacterial medications and rising microbial virulence. Traditional indigenous plant-based medicines and therapies, unlike the biologically aggressive compounds created by our nature-dominating society, are nourishing, strengthening, cleansing, and rejuvenating, and promote individual, social, and ecological equilibrium. (338-341)

We live on a planet that belongs to bacteria. They are the most abundant organisms on earth, whose collective weight is greater than all other forms of life combined. The human body is inhabited by highly intelligent microbial communities composed of hundreds of types of bacteria, viruses, yeasts, and other organisms, in unimaginable numbers. On one square inch of intestine there are more microbes than humans on the planet. A trillion bacteria live on our skin, 10 billion reside in our mouth, and 10 billion are flushed down the toilet after every bowel movement. Over 300 different types of bacteria swim in the digestive tract. Overall, about 100 trillion individual organisms consider each of our bodies as their home. Almost all of them live a harmonious synergistic existence with the others, and with us.

These organisms play an important role in sustaining our health. The microbes of the digestive tract help digest different classes of foods, manufacture vitamins needed by the body, and break down chemical toxins. By attaching themselves to the intestinal wall and competing for nutrients, they form a protective colony against invading organisms. They produce natural antibiotic substances, stimulate the production of antibodies to fight infection, and destroy pathogenic organisms. We owe our health, digestive capacity, and immunity to the complex intelligence of the microbial communities within us.

---

[2] Marigpa translates as spiritual ignorance (Crow 373).

"Three basic causes of disease have been given in Ayurveda," [says Dr. Singh, a doctor of Ayurvedic medicine]. "The first is the improper combination of our senses with the sense objects, that is, excessive, deficient, or perverted. The second cause is if you do something against your conscience, your innate knowledge. And the third cause is time factors, like the seasons. Now, in all these three, where do the bacteria come in? The bacteria will grow only if these conditions are conducive. So the emphasis is on the field, the proper soil, the proper climate, rather than on the seed...."

Louis Pasteur was the father of microbiology and the originator of modern science's germ theory. His ideas about germs being the causative agents of disease were widely debated by scientists of his day. At the end of his life, Pasteur expressed his final views, which were the same as Ayurveda's. "The microbe is nothing," he declared, "the terrain everything." (342-343)

Although the Ayurvedic pharmacopoeia contains numerous botanical drugs with highly effective antibiotic properties, developing the body's resistance by restoring equilibrium with the terrain of tissues and humors is the primary goal of treatment, while subduing microbial toxins is secondary; most formulations for infectious febrile conditions simultaneously "attack" pathogens and "support" vitality. The emerging pharmaceutical industry in the West, however, found the pursuit of a "magic bullet" that could simply eradicate germs far more lucrative than preventive measures such as lifestyle modifications and enhancement of immunity using natural methods. Four antibiotic generations later the long-term consequences of this "attacking" philosophy are now appearing in the microbial kingdom....

Under the influence of antibiotics, the weakest strains of bacteria die off and the hardiest mutate to survive. These increasingly virulent strains pass on new genetic information to their offspring, and more powerful substances are required to control each succeeding generation. Common types of bacteria have mutated into a wide variety of new forms, appearing in outbreaks of "superinfections" and medically resistant forms of old diseases such as tuberculosis and gonorrhea. While strengthening unwanted organisms, antibiotics also weaken the beneficial ones by eradicating the healthy microbial communities of the body. The combined results are decreased immunity and vitality, susceptibility to over-growth and reinfection by invasive microbes, and accumulation of disease-promoting toxic residues. Using Chinese medical terminology, these effects can be described as "treating the stem while weakening the root." This symptomatic approach does not address causative factors....

If scientists had deliberately set out to radically alter the global microbial environment, they could not have found a better way to do so. In the space of a few decades, we have planted the seeds of virulent disorder in the microbial soil; now those seeds are coming to fruition, bringing the end of the antibiotic era. The fundamental shortsightedness of the allopathic paradigm — overlooking and underestimating the far-reaching repercussions of biochemical interference with nature's complex intelligence — is more apparent now than ever. The painful lesson to be learned from medically created diseases is that therapies which compromise human ecology must at least be supported, if not replaced whenever possible, by treatments which strengthen resistance. As modern drugs lose their effectiveness, the spiritual wisdom of the physician-sages and their vitalistic methods of healing will once again play a central role in medical practice. A holistic paradigm emphasizing harmony and compatibility with other forms of life will deepen in the psyche of the world, accompanied by a renaissance of traditional plant-based healing systems such as Ayurveda. (343-345)

> The myriad diseases affecting humanity arise from a small number of underlying causes: malnutrition, weakened immunity, biotoxicity, and microbial pathogenesis. These fundamental roots of sickness are primarily the results of ecological and social degradation, which is created by human behaviors originating within the mind" (350-351).
>
> ... Mindfulness of the composite nature and therefore impermanent basis of existence decreases our false sense of selfhood and inspires the "wisdom of not possessing" by helping us feel how we are part of everything, yet utterly devoid of any substantiality. This biological spirituality, and the sattvic view[3] of life it awakens, is the antidote to marigpa's greed and violence, and the damage they have done to the earth....
>
> ... Perhaps the most valuable contribution Ayurveda has to offer the world is its definition of health: equilibrium among the humors, tissues, transformations, and wastes; and happiness of mind, senses, and soul. True health is the result of living harmoniously with the forces of nature, and the fruit of a culture's flowering spiritual maturity. Long-term ecological equilibrium, the global foundation of individual health, can be brought about only through sattvic consciousness guiding a society that loves, respects, and nurtures human, plant, and animal life. This is Bhaisajyaguru's kingdom of Sudarshan, a vision of the flourishing natural wealth bestowed upon civilizations that practice compassionate Dharma for the benefit of all living beings.[4]
>
> Like a mirror of our Buddha-nature, Sudarshan reflects humanity's capacity to create thriving, enlightened cultures. Integrating universal truth, ecology, and medicine, the iconographic symbolism of the Medicine Buddha's mandala contains layers of teachings to assist us in becoming skilled and gentle guardians of the earth's healing treasures.... Sudarshan is the beauty, health, and happiness which await us, when the human mind has assumed its proper place in the pattern of Creation, and our lives once again follow the ancient rhythms of peaceful coexistence with nature. (352-353)
>
> Beautiful to Behold is luxuriously endowed with trees of all kinds.[5] Sandalwood and camphor infuse the air with sensuous energizing fragrance, aquillaria gives precious oil of oud, willowlike branches of pepper trees offer their spicy berries, cinnamon exudes its sweet pungence, and towering neem provide bitter antibiotics from the leaves and bark. All types of myrobalans grow plentifully, as well as sour amla, the master rejuvenator. Pomegranates and other fruits burst with ripe juices, essential oils, and medicinal seeds. The caroblike pods of cassia trees dangle in the breeze; pines, cedars, and junipers release their aromatic breath; rhododendrons paint impressionistic scenes with pastel flowers.

---

[3] Sattvic translates as that which is good for everyone. (Crow 263)

[4] Dharma in Ayurvedic philosophy expresses that which is both beneficial and necessary for one. (Crow 262)

[5] Beautiful to Behold is the translation of Sudarshan which is the mythical world of Bhaisajyaguru — one of several physician bodhisattvas or universal Buddhas (Crow 22). The symbolic meaning behind Sudarshan is: "enlightened consciousness governing a sacred society, which lives harmoniously within a flourishing and healthy natural environment" (Crow 332-333). And above you have just read another description of Sudarshan as the "beauty, health and happiness which await us . . ." (Crow 353).

Appendix B

The wondrous trees that once graced the earth made a way for human life to emerge, and they continue, even as we destroy them, to silently sustain us. Trees feed us, cure us, protect us, and bless us with an abundance of resources. They bring rains, yet keep them from becoming destructive, hold the soil, regenerate its fertility, purify the toxins we spread across the land, give us oxygen, and cleanse the sky. Because of trees, all beings can drink pure water, and breathe. As we destroy the trees, springs stop flowing, wells run dry, vegetation withers, animals disappear, storms intensify, and desert sands begin to arrive. If there is to be a home for coming generations, nations must replant their trees and care for their arboreal heritage. (353-354)

All plants use their toxin-transforming physiology to purify the earth's elements. Many kinds of trees, shrubs, grasses, and herbaceous plants are being effectively utilized to cleanse the poisons we have thoughtlessly dumped in every part of the globe. Certain species, such as alpine penncress and datura, hyperaccumulate toxic metals and chemicals, either converting them into less dangerous forms or concentrating the substances for further reprocessing. Poplars are being used to decontaminate soils ruined by dry-cleaning chemicals and petroleum products. Sunflowers bred to absorb strontium and cesium are being tested as a way of neutralizing the radiation around Chernobyl, and water hyacinths are used in sewage treatment. As the chemical, metallic, and radioactive wastes of modern culture multiply and their pathogenic effects increase in the population, phytoremediation will become one of humankind's most important livelihoods. Crops with specialized curative powers are appearing on military bases, around nuclear plants, and over chemical spills, bringing us one step closer to the pure land of Sudarshan.

By taking care of plants, we will in turn be cared for. As sickness, hunger and chaos come in rising waves, the reintegration of civilization and the botanical kingdom will become an increasingly urgent necessity, and the fertile ground from which Sudarshan could emerge. A collective awakening to our dependency on the plant kingdom for nourishment, medicine, clothing, and shelter may catalyze societies to abandon obsolete, dangerous and wasteful habits, and begin a new era of botanical stewardship. In urban gardens, agroforests, and eco-villages, families once isolated and estranged from nature's rhythms could again participate in the plants' eternal cycles of germination and fruition and gradually reenter the stream of harmonious existence. . . . As community forests and garden cities flourish on every continent, nations may begin resembling those in the pure lands of Beautiful to Behold, where devic caretakers labor peacefully around the jeweled palace of enlightenment. If we skillfully sow seeds of ecological compassion, we will harvest abundant blessings. (354-355)

The healing of humanity's ancient wounds and the rebirth of Dharmic culture rests upon ecological renewal. Environmental restoration is a unifying purpose that brings together families of diverse racial, ethnic, economic, and religious backgrounds in a common struggle against the threat of biospheric collapse. . . . As communities and nations join hands in mutual concern for plants, animals, and coming generations, the long history of inflicting pain on others may cease, and true spirituality reawaken (356).

Appendix C: Excerpts from Tachyon Energy[1]

As we come to more personally, intuitively, and eventually measurably (or at least as measurable as quantum physics[2] and mechanics are or can be) know ourselves and our energetic composition and that of the ethers, we will then have at our behest an exquisitely richer understanding of health and causation. And it is into this realm of the extraordinarily possible, that I would then see us positioning our use and our understanding of tachyon energy and the sacred funnels of our subtle organizing energy fields:

integrated tachyon theory of healing

The use of tachyon energy... empowers us to evolve through dynamic chaos to the next level of order, rather than getting mired in stuck chaos.

Tachyon energy significantly helps us to make that move more rapidly. With the use of Tachyon, we are presenting not only a full holistic model of healing, but a process by which we can each move toward radiant health. In this state there is a free flow of energy through the entire body, mind, and spirit that results in a continuous experience of well being in every moment independent of the outer world. The human energy system is a dynamic system. We must be continually supplied with energy, and a substantial source of the energy needed by humans is assimilated through the subtle energy systems of the body. One of the subtle energetic systems is called the chakra system.

The chakras are a series of vortices located in seven regions of the physical body: crown or top of head; third eye, located between the eyes of the brow; throat; heart; solar plexus; sexual area; and perineal area, located near the end of the coccyx

---

[1] Please see *Sources Cited* under Wagner and Cousens.

[2] I've been looking for a reasonable place to slip in the following snippet on quantum physics and suppose here serves as well as any. Hence, let us notice that quantum physics doesn't eclipse or even compromise Newtonian physics. We need both on the energetic continuum of physics. Quantum extends to the *nano* end of the scale with a specificity Newtonian physics can't access and doesn't need to engineer a bridge (Phillips, please see *Sources Cited*, "Continuum of Physics.")

and one inch in front of the anus.[3]

In nature everything has its own self-contained vertical energy structure. This vertical structure, although independent, is also interconnected with all local vertical structures, humans and earth. When we are born our chakra system resembles this vertical energy system. It is vertical and connected to All That Is. Currently, when people grow up in our society, the chakra system loses its verticality and alignment with the ordered flow of life-force energy.... The horizontal energy system is fragmented, and normally all but the crown and root chakra become horizontal.... In the process of becoming horizontal, we lose part of our natural connection with the energetic flow of nature. The horizontal shift decreases the quantity of energy flowing through the chakra system and therefore into the body.

This decreased energy in our body creates a subtle shift in which we unconsciously begin to seek to increase our energy from outside forces. There are several healthy ways to enhance our energy, including nurturing our bodies with love foods, pure water, sunlight, meditation, and taking in the elemental energies of the air, earth, water, and sunlight. Association with like-minded people is also very helpful.

In our social world there are several unhealthy ways of enhancing our energy. One common way to get energy is to unconsciously steal it from other people. This is normally done as destructive competition or plain usurpation. These practices are most obviously seen in the business world. For example, if two business men or women enter into a discussion, each presents his or her case in a way that seeks to make them superior to the other, usurping the other's energy. This process goes back and forth until there is a winner and a loser. The loser is depleted; the winner is energized. The loser may begin to scan the horizon for the next situation. If it isn't found, then his or her family may become unfortunate providers of the needed energy. And what if the spouse also is drained? The cycle is unfortunate and unnecessary. When this is extrapolated to the global level, it supplies the social theory to explain the resistance to global peace and it also serves as the source of all planetary atrocities.

The need to feel superior and to dominate an individual or a society is a dominator's way of increasing energy. This is shortsighted because it creates and strengthens a block for the natural flow of the life force. Dominators may appear to increase energy for one person or one type of society, but it ultimately decreases it for everyone. The reason for this is that the energy is stolen and not in a natural continual flow that connects the person or society to All That Is. Usurping energy from others is associated with a dominator approach, versus the partnership way of being in the world, which adds to each person's energy. (3-5)

Through the use of specialized Tachyonized™ materials and techniques it is possible to shift from a needy, horizontal energetic system to a vertically aligned partnership system of being connected to the divine source of All That Is. When one becomes vertical, one receives a constant flow of energy feeding the emotional, mental, physical, and spiritual bodies. This is our natural way of being. When a business person is vertical, he or she is in a partnership/cooperative mode that enhances everyone's energy. This ultimately eliminates the need to win at the expense of others. Such people tap into the natural order/chaos/order process, thus allowing the creation of balanced solutions that work for everyone. These remarkable individuals

---

[3] Next esoteric information guides us to consider twelve or thirteen chakras.

Appendix C

become icons in their cycle of peers as someone who is always present, fair, and respectful. These individuals, by their vertical nature, never deplete a situation. They are a source of harmonizing energy, healing and balancing the world by just being. They become natural leaders in the movement toward peace and harmony, regardless of their profession.

The healing or evolution of chaos into order creates harmony. We may work with people and even compete in a way that is enhancing and synergistically improving what we are doing based on mutual growth by valuing each other's ideas. This actually creates a healing or another level of order in terms of how to be in the world. The understanding of order/chaos/order is not just on the physical plane of dis-ease, but clearly includes the mental, emotional, and spiritual planes. By reestablishing our vertical connection, we can move out of domination into harmonic partnership without taking energy from each other but instead adding energy to each other. This shift helps the move to a higher level of order.

As we go a little deeper into the paradigm of holistic health we see that the harmony and healing of the body, the emotions, and the mental and spiritual levels are based on an energy source that is primordial to our existence. Healing at every level is very dependent on tapping into the primordial cosmic energy, which is the source of existence. So the deepest level of holistic healing, and even of maintenance and rejuvenation, is made possible by our ability to tap into this cosmic energy that energizes and creates the form of all material existence as we know it. It is at this deeper level that we can begin to appreciate and integrate the meaning of Tachyon energy as the new paradigm in holistic healing.

Tachyon energy is the bridge to higher and higher amplitudes of cosmic energy that can power our healing, rejuvenation, and return to verticality. This is really the secret of the whole thing. It is the secret to spontaneous healing; it is the secret to all such miracles. We all have the potential to link into or directly attune to this higher primordial energy. Some people may call the energy God; some people may call it cosmic energy; science calls it Zero-Point energy. . . .

In order to understand integration of the physical and the pure energy world, we need to develop a theory of how material existence comes into being. Such great people as Einstein and Nikola Tesla spent a lot of time on this subject, and many of their theories are included in the new physics and quantum mechanics thinking. The theory basically states that our body exists "as a precipitation out of an invisible unbounded totality of perfect order." This unbounded perfect order has been called by several names: virtual energy, Zero-Point energy, vacuum state, or ether are some examples. . . .

To further understand this primordial energy it really helps to merge science and holistic healing by using the language that science uses in talking about it. So we will now talk about this primordial energy as science does by calling it Zero-Point energy. (5-7)

The world of science has been proving that matter is simply the condensation of a vibrating universal subtle energy substratum, which is the virtual state otherwise known as the zero-point energy. In the production of matter, zero-point energy simply condenses into Tachyon energy, which is then converted into frequencies by the SOEFs (subtle organizing energy fields), creating all varieties of forms. . . .

As the condensation of a vibrating universal subtle energy substratum, or a virtual state or vacuum in a matrix of time and space, matter is made of particular forms and densities of energy. In other words, matter is the manifest structure of all of nature and the laws governing all physical phenomena. In spiritual terminology, *pure consciousness, cosmic energy, and universal prana* are terms analogous to this perfectly orderly manifested state. SOEFs are an attempt to describe how this precipitation from subtle energy to material form takes place and how it is ordered.

Science calls the potential energy, which fills the cosmos, zero-point energy. Zero point exists prior to the materialization of an object....

Zero-point energy is omnipresent; it permeates the entire universe. It also exists in infinite quantity; that is, it can never be exhausted. There are three characteristics of zero-point energy, which are of paramount significance for us in our world: The first is that zero-point energy contains all potential. Within zero-point energy is everything needed to create perfect form. The second characteristic of zero-point energy is that it is formless and unmanifested. The third characteristic of zero-point energy is that it is omnipresent in the universe. In summary, zero-point energy is omnipresent in the universe, it permeates everything, it exists in infinite quantity, it is completely inexhaustible, and it contains all the potentials of perfect form. (7-8)

The first stepping-down of this formless, unmanifested zero-point energy is into Tachyon energy.... The energy then continues to be stepped-down and patterned into material forms. It also interacts in various energetic ways with material forms. This interplay of research and theory provided the Subtle Organizing Energy Field matrix for Dr. Cousens' theory as outlined in his book:

> ...these are fields, which both create and energize the template form of living systems. SOEFs exist throughout all aspects of the energetic continuum. As SOEFs emerge out of the virtual state, they are capable of organizing on any level of the human body, from cellular structure to the organ systems, and even to subtle bodies. These SOEFs resonate with the unlimited virtual state energy, transferring it through various step-down systems that eventually transude it into the energy fields of the human body. The SOEFs thus resonate with and energize the body-mind complex.
>
> Zero-point energy is omnipresent; thus we are always resonating to some extent with this cosmic energy. Most of the time we have only indirect or brief experiences of this, but at certain stages of spiritual evolution it is possible to experience this resonance in direct attunement, consistently and consciously. For many, this sort of experience first happens in meditation. As we become more aware of and resonant with this virtual energy state, our minds merge and identify with this awareness as the unchanging truth and the reality of our existence. The resonance becomes part of our conscious awareness in our everyday activities. Eventually, it becomes a continual awareness and attunement with the cosmic energy. This is known as cosmic consciousness.
>
> By increasing the tachyon energy in our lives, we directly increase our resonance with the zero-point energy. We therefore improve all levels of body, emotion, mind and spiritual health and enhance the process of moving to higher levels of order in our lives. This accelerates the healing and spiritual evolutionary process for ourselves.[4]

There is another important ramification of zero-point energy physics that is relevant to our new holistic health par-

Appendix C

adigm. It is called the theory of conservation of energy. This theory explains how entropy can be reversed and biological transmutation can take place in the human system without breaking any fundamental laws. With this theory as one of our building blocks, we are able to develop a new holistic healing model — a model that explains how the unlimited formless zero-point energy condenses into tachyon energy form, which is then converted into specific frequencies by the SOEFs. This energy is transduced into the human body in a way that reverses entropy and therefore reverses aging....

... This continual process of the SOEFs converting Tachyon energy into the needed frequencies... continues all the way down through the energetic continuum. It continues until the perfect form is ultimately reached, whether it is a human being or any other form that we know of. Tachyon energy is the binding energy of the universe and is responsible for the creation of all forms on the planet. Tachyon energy is the key element in the flow of energy from the infinitely formless all the way down to the perfect form. This flow we call the energetic continuum.

As with all forms in our slower-than-light universe, SOEFs cannot exceed the speed of light. This is a very important point. Our world is a world of form, so the only way for us to interface with formless zero-point energy is through tachyon. The condensation of zero-point energy moves from the unlimited formless zero-point energy into tachyon energy, which is the step prior to slowing to the speed of light. The tachyon energy at this point is moving faster than the speed of light and is prior to all frequencies. Tachyon has no frequency, and as a faster-than-light energy obviously has no spin, vibration, or oscillation yet contains the potential of all frequencies. From a scientific point of view, only frequencies manifest a spin or oscillation. Tachyon energy is the energetic bridge between Zero-Point energy and the SOEFs. The SOEFs are in direct communion with tachyon energy on all levels. It is through the SOEFs that the tachyon energy is converted into all levels of frequencies and forms.

Tachyon energy is therefore the critical factor which energizes the SOEFs. So the more Tachyon energy we bring into our olives, the more energized and therefore organized are our SOEFs. The energizing of the SOEFs is what creates health and rejuvenation because it reverses entropy, or aging. When tachyon energy is free-flowing, we have an endless source of energy to rebuild and maintain our SOEFs, so we continually reverse entropy. This explains how the body can, in effect, become a "faster-than-light energy" conduit, since we are linked to the unlimited zero-point energy as our ultimate source of energy. As a result, the body-mind complex becomes more clear and balanced in spiritual evolution, and it becomes an increasingly better transducer and conductor of energy. As this happens, the body is able to store and transmit greater and greater amounts of this higher energy. This process can account for some of the many miracles said to occur in the presence of spiritual masters. For example, spontaneous healing occurred when people simply touched the robe of Jesus. We now understand that there was a flow of this pure cosmic or God energy into people that reorganized and reenergized their SOEFs, allowing the dis-ease processes to be reversed. People's faith allowed them to draw and be receptive to the healing energy.

SOEFs have both form and energy. They can hold, gain, lose, resonate with, transduce, and transmit energy. Because

---

[✦] Gabriel Cousens, M.D. quoting in Tachyon Energy: A New Paradigm in Holistic Healing (8-9) from his book Spiritual Nutrition and the Rainbow Diet.

of this, they are different from Rupert Sheldrake's hypotheses of morphogenic fields described in *A New Science of Life*. His morphogenic fields are concerned only with form; they are neither a type of matter nor a type of energy. Sheldrake's description of the morphogenic fields and his brilliant hypothesis of formative causation describes the form aspect of SOEFs beautifully. According to Sheldrake, morphogenic fields play a causal role in the development and maintenance of the forms of systems at all levels. Sheldrake uses the term "morphic unit" as a way to describe the sub-units in a system, that is, a morphic unit for protons; another for atoms, water molecules, and muscle cells; and another for organs such as kidneys. The higher morphic fields coordinate the interplay, organization, and pattern of the smaller morphic units. Like the SOEFs, these morphogenic fields correspond to the potential state of a developing system and are present before it materializes into its final form. (8-11)

Appendix D: Excerpts from *Earth in Ascension*[1]

As we come to understand and to know in the most interior and precious parts of ourselves that there is truly nothing to forgive, that all is indeed in divine right order and timing, and that there are only synchronicities, and an exquisitely dense veil of them, life and our relationship with her alters forever. Already, for some this veil is less hidden and carries an intermittent vibration of iridescence, connection, and delight. For others, it is rarely noticed and even then, usually attributed to coincidence without inspiring curiosity or touching ethereal memories of presence, continuity, and blessings woven of opportunity and choreography. But with time, as we all move more profoundly into these understandings, judging and the either/ors of duality along with the paradigms of polarity all shift gently out of focus and out of consciousness and are replaced by the both/ands of fifth and sixth dimensionality's unconditional love and unconditional compassion.

Let us further pursue this Shift as we examine more closely these blessing and pivotal years as we draw closer and closer to the majesty of the Ages Shifting as chronicled in Mayan, Incan, Andean, New Age and numerous other texts and resources (Essene, You Are Becoming 14):

[considerations]

It becomes very clear that many dolphins and whales have brains that are superior to humans, brains and bodies that are more highly evolved. However, they have chosen lives of service and sacrifice, absorbing human negativity to help ease the overwhelming burdens on Mother Earth. Oh, the heart pain that is felt for the animals as thousands of years of human subjugation and mishandling seem to pass through the cellular memory of each person. But as quickly as those thoughts come in, they flow out again. The collective consciousness begins clearing its RNA/DNA patterning. After many ages the

---

[1] Please see *Sources Cited* under Clark.

new humanity is becoming filled with a sense of loving obligation, realizing they must be custodial guardians caring for and nurturing the animal kingdom.

Suddenly it is so apparent! Every single subatomic particle on and in this planet is necessary to her balance. Every system was slowly and deliberately created to work in harmony with everything else. Each person's mind wonders how humans could have deceived themselves into believing that the continuous rape of Earth would have no repercussions. Could it be that humans have thought of themselves as being separate from Source for so long that they have also believed that everything else is separate? Nothing could be further from the truth. It has been said that the flutter of a butterfly's wings in the Pacific can cause a hurricane in the Atlantic. It is critical to Earth's survival that every human become aware that all aspects of Earth have consciousness — from the oceans and the trees to the energy vibrations of which they are made.

It is no longer acceptable to participate in a world bent on amassing material goods at the expense of all the other kingdoms which are as much a part of the Earth as humans are. . . .

Then the focus shifts to those who really care, the ones who truly love the land. They can be found in every nation. These people feel deep concern for the growing problems and wish to help in any way they can. There is the thought of banding together to protest and to fight the injustices of the world. But immediately there is a strong reaction from all the kingdoms: that reaction is love! Collectively, they send the message that it is no longer appropriate to protest or to fight for what is considered right. That has been tried for thousands of years and the only result has been more fighting.

Now is the time to think with and act from the heart. No judgment. No violence. The only responsible reaction is to surround the negative actions with love. Once a person gains this perspective, he operates from a place of inner peace in which every outward action is the result of the inward knowingness of pure love. Others want to know his secret, wondering what he is doing that is making him so happy, and they want to be in his presence so that the tranquility and joy will radiate to their beings.

This experience has enlarged each person's vision. For a moment the vistas of life as they really exist were opened, and it was one of the few occasions when mind and ego did not distort reality. At that time the basic patterning in the RNA/DNA was transformed from separatism to unity.

Humanity has moved beyond relying on ego for survival. It was ego that long ago created the sense of duality. The first stage of human evolvement was, according to the ancient teachings, "Man, know thyself," and that could be accomplished only through separation and egoism. Now it is important to recognize with all senses that the majority of people have completed their first great step.

The next stage of human evolution is the integration of the soul. It is in this initiation that humans must learn the other ancient teaching: "Man, forget thyself." It is the dawn of the age of brotherhood when humans exist in loving relationship with the living and the nonliving, the great and the minute. People sense that each of them is one unit of the great collective. Every deed and action begins to be carried out from the perspective of how others will be affected. Most humans are realizing during this period that God is within as well as without. They are discovering their God-like abilities. This is the knowledge that will bring the thousand years of peace. Following very swiftly upon that stage is the third stage, during which the spirit of humanity becomes fully integrated. Then the fusion of all of consciousness will be complete. People will have stopped asking God for favors in their prayers and they will have stopped trying to be God-like, for they will truly know they are God. It will have become impossible to see anything as being outside of God. From this new perspective, everything that happens is either love or a lesson in love. (67-70)

new perspectives

Earth's population is witnessing a greater period of change in a shorter period of time than even the Spiritual Hierarchy of the planet had envisioned....

The greatest change will be in consciousness....

C. Jung's term, "collective unconscious," refers to energy that is made up of attitudes, beliefs, interpretations and feelings of the world's population. This collective energy defines what is real and what is not real for the people existing in a particular time and place. In the past, race, nationality, gender, social status, religion and education have been some of the aspects that have developed localized characteristics of consciousness. When these various facets of reality are added together, they form the collective unconscious.

At this time the collective is not only rapidly changing but it is also rapidly expanding. The drug experimentation of the sixties immediately altered reality for the entire planet. There has been continuous experimentation with drugs over the past fifty years, especially under the auspices of governmental research. In addition to artificially induced altered states of consciousness, many "normal" people have become interested in meditation, pranic breathing$_1$ or, more recently, Holotropic Breathwork,$_2$ jogging, and yoga, not to forget hypnosis and the many forms of release therapy. All these and many more take the practitioner into other realities and other realms of consciousness.

Many parallel realities exist on Earth now. Most are separate or distinct but, like the ages and the dimensions, they overlap and interpenetrate one another. (71-72)

The subject of extraterrestrials provides a good example of parallel realities. There are still people who believe no life exists beyond the Earth, and that is their reality. Others have read books and seen television reports about alien life forms and believe they could exist. Still another group of people have seen spacecraft for themselves and have perhaps even been aboard a ship....

It will be understood shortly that a group of humans have agreed to continue life on the third-dimensional level with the help of alien beings from several different planetary systems. Overwhelmingly negative information has been spread about this project, but the experiment was designed to improve existing races through the hybridization of the species.

For example, the Grays are reported to have become unable to experience emotions due to the atrophying of their emotional bodies through disuse and also to have lost the ability to reproduce. In contrast, many humans are very emotional and are reproducing irresponsibly. This mutually agreed-upon project is intended to create a race with the advanced abilities of the Grays and the positive attributes of humans. Those who have agreed to take part in the experiment realized they were not yet ready to move into the fifth dimension on Earth's timetable, so they agreed to this grand experiment in another third-dimensional situation. For many years these special people have been learning to adjust to life on spaceships in preparation for their journey to their new home planet. In truth, the abductees are pioneers who have agreed to settle a New Earth, having made that decision at higher levels of being. Aliens involved in the project believe they are helping humanity as well as themselves; it is not a purely selfish venture as people are often led to believe. (73-74)

Many of the extraterrestrials involved in this project are extremely concerned about human well-being. One of the considerate and compassionate plans they have for their human families is to provide surroundings as familiar as possible. To create another Earth, it is necessary to gather plant and animal specimens for future adaptation (75).

During the coming years, the true meaning of duality and illusion will become increasingly apparent as humanity begins to experience two very opposite realities. For one segment of the population, there will be increasing chaos in which nothing seems to work and life is a constant struggle to survive. It will be impossible for those experiencing utter confusion and disorder to see beyond the world of illusion — which they are creating. They will believe everyone is out to get them. It will seem very apparent to them that they are about to lose their jobs, their homes, their money and their partners. Each day will seem to bring greater fear. They will have difficulty sleeping, and the food they eat will not be properly digested. A combination of headaches, chest pains, backaches and digestive problems including ulcers will manifest periodically. As they believe the boss, the car salesperson and the government are out to get them, so it will be. Their fears will become their realities.

Existing temporarily in this scene will be another picture of reality altogether. A second group of humanity is discovering greater joy, deeper peace and an inexplicable optimism about the future. Each day brings a growing sense of destiny. These people know their time is coming. They realize there are the times and events they came to witness. Personal and global disasters seem to pass right by these individuals. They feel as though they are living in a protective bubble. This group is not preoccupied with individual survival. Rather, their great need is to be of service. They are willing to work for the benefit of all and are directing energy toward the healing of the planet. More than any other attribute, they are learning to be flexible and to face whatever circumstance develops. It is easy to understand that the distance between the two groups is growing greater with each passing day. (77)

These images are only probable realities. There is no need for a disaster of any magnitude if humanity desires to move forward with Earth in her ascension. But there is an absolute necessity to stop any fear-based thoughts regarding the possible futures. Those who are able to create the reality of a smooth transition should meditate on and visualize this daily, alone or in groups. All imaging of a best-case scenario outcome will produce great benefits for the entire planet.

... [T]he process begins on an individual basis and as a result of a gradual awakening. The first step involves changing the way people view their experience and how they react to those situations....

As humans become more open in their thinking, they automatically become less judgmental, which leads to being more accepting and unconditionally loving. (81)

As a person begins to create a more loving, less stressful life, his mental body rises up from the denser subplanes. The subatomic particles that make up this body are actually able to carry more Light (83).

… The more time individuals spend in joy, the more quickly their atoms fill with Light. The Light particles that fill the mental and emotional bodies influence the amount of Light the etheric and physical bodies can contain (85).

This is a unique and historical time to be living on Earth.… When the population has reached critical mass by raising their vibrations and becoming spirit-conscious…, the remainder of the inhabitants and the planet will transform instantly!

What unbelievable joy! Is it any wonder thousands of "unwanted" babies are flooding the planet? Everyone who possibly can wants to take part in the experience.…

… Unfathomable numbers of souls have incarnated on Earth since the beginning, so all could not be present at this time; there simply is not enough space. Those who are here now are considered fortunate by all those watching from the different dimensions. This is some indication of how extraordinary these times are. Relax and enjoy the ride. It is just going to get better. (86-87)

It is time to remember that life on this planet has been an experiment. Many souls created bodies to experience density and the material world; they chose to investigate separation and duality. Now they are on the journey home. The most difficult work is behind and the glorious work lies ahead. The separation ends as people awaken to their oneness with All That Is — not just here, not just now, but everywhere and for all time. The more each can identify with his or her individual uniqueness, the more it is possible to appreciate being totally one. Individuals are really Sparks of the Creator who is the Source of all Light: "I and my Father are One" or, in New Thought, "I Am one with the Source." This is all very beautiful and very esoteric but it is time to learn the details of personal ascension. (91)

discovering wellness

Once people awaken from their present limited thinking, they will realize their bodies have never descended from perfection; they will see the illusion of past limited thinking and begin recreating their perfect selves. Most illness originates in the emotional body or the mental body. From there is goes into (infects) the etheric body. The last body to become ill is the physical body.…

As people become emotionally healthier and more spiritually attuned, it will be easier to be totally healed and to remain in perfect health. It is important to remember that healing the body is one thing, but if the emotional, mental and spiritual problems that caused the illness are not resolved, the disease will recur.…

Many individuals on their path are trying to treat their physical bodies better than they ever have before in this lifetime, yet they suffer from aches, pains, flu and various symptoms for which no doctor can determine a cause. The good news is that physical symptoms are an indication that the body's vibrational level is increasing. The higher vibrations actually shake old stagnant energy out of the organs, muscles and tissues just like a dog shaking off water. Even though these high vibrations are causing more aches and pains now, eventually all the discomfort will disappear. Any kind of bodywork such as massage or energy therapy can be very helpful in moving the stuck energy out of the body more quickly.

All the physical bodies are being restructured at a cellular level while the other bodies are changing vibrationally. (96-97)

physical symptoms common to the ascension process

There are quite a number of physical changes occurring in human bodies because the species is evolving. Those who have not yet been affected can expect to notice symptoms in the near future.

1. Ringing in the ears
    a. Messages are actually being sent in tonal patterns.
    b. People are becoming more aware of the sounds of individual organs. In the future, it will be possible to detect if the heart or gall bladder or liver is stressed because they will be out of harmony with the rest of the body's tones.
    c. People are becoming more sensitive to the electronic waves and frequencies which penetrate most areas of the globe. These high-pitched sounds can become very loud and distracting at times.

2. Heart palpitations occur as the heart restructures in alignment with a higher vibration. The muscles of the heart have always been striated vertcally, as are all organs that are involuntary. Recently more and more of the heart's muscles are becoming striated horizontally, which means that in the future, people will be responsible for the action of their hearts. Advanced yogis always know how to control their hearts and other organs.

3. A change in eyesight
    a. Blurring of vision occurs as the eyes restructure.
    b. People think they see someone beyond their range of vision, just over their shoulder. In truth, they are seeing into another dimension and actually seeing an etheric being or spirit.
    c. Some individuals see waterfalls of light and halos around electric lights. This is terrifying for those who know someone with glaucoma, but the truth is they are beginning to see into other dimensions. In the beginning people seldom see straight ahead into other planes. Instead, they see into other planes, peripherally, or from the side.
    d. Many people, especially those in their twenties and younger, see the colorful auras around everyone and everything.

4. Hot and cold flashes regardless of age and gender, are the result of metabolic changes. This unpleasantness can be greatly alleviated by rapping gently below the notch in the throat at the thymus gland. People also find it helpful to request that their guides regulate their metabolism while they are sleeping.

5. Experiencing chills throughout the body occurs when someone is imparting information. This is the new way the body has chosen to let individuals become informed of their own truth. It also allows a person to adjust the frequency of his or her own vibration to that of another, which becomes increasingly important as the masters come here to teach humanity.

6. Difficulty with memory sometimes occurs, leading people to wonder if they are losing their minds, because they seem to be forgetting more information than they are remembering. This is happening because useless data are being deleted from individual memory banks, especially the untruths programmed during school years. It allows areas of the brain to be used more efficiently.

7. A sense of loss and a feeling of being overwhelmed with sadness can fill the emotions, usually with good reason. Lifelong friends and even family might have become distant. It is increasingly difficult to find something in common. Serious illness is affecting individuals or their loved ones. Many people are losing their jobs and homes. So much is changing in such a short time. This is not punishment; it is happening so that people will move into the areas of service they came into this life to perform.

8. Food cravings, especially for sweets. It is comforting to know that meditation and psychic work use far more of the brain's blood sugar than do normal activities. Physical bodies require far less food than most people think they do, but they require greater amounts of purified water. Fewer medications, drugs, hormones and supplements are needed now, and many people are aware of an increasing sensitivity to artificial products. Drugs, alcohol, food and sex mask what must be faced in life now.

All these symptoms seem to come and go along with the aches and pains as old energy blocks work their way to the surface. (97-100)

[who are we as human beings?]

The human was designed with enormous care.... Individual spirits specifically and precisely constructed perfect bodies for this particular mission. The human body is still in its outer wrapping, giving only a hint of its contents, but the season is fast approaching when humans will be able to open the package and discover their true beauty, beauty that has never been seen in a mirror. Each individual must unwrap his own gift and awaken to reconnect with his higher self.... Once that has been done, the Light will be shared throughout the planet (104).

... [There] is a recognition that all people are one, in spite of their individuality.

The feeling of being family fills people with even more Light. As they look out into the distance, they watch in amazement as their lights connect with thousands of other Lights. Together, humanity appears to be creating a grid of Light on the surface of the planet. As more links occur, the Lights flash and glisten even brighter. Some people send out rays of a particular hue that stretch out and connect with similar rays. As cobalt blue joins cobalt blue, and magenta unites with magenta, a sensation arises in the heart center that makes a person aware that he is connecting with a member of his soul family.

As the Light grids radiate out to distant stars and planets, sensations of warmth and belonging flood a person's body, and he realizes that he has just reconnected to those distant realms which are also his home. Next, he becomes aware that Light and love are flowing out through his feet down to the heart of Mother Earth as he expresses his gratitude in a fifth-dimensional way....

A tranquil realization floods the consciousness; there is a knowing that nothing on this plane of reality will revert to the way it was. Everything in the world has been shifted a little farther into the next dimension. (63)

...A drop of water removed from the ocean has very little value, but as part of the ocean it is a powerful force. The same principle applies to love. Every little act of kindness, every loving glance or touch, every reassuring word becomes a part of the vast ocean of cosmic love, instantly connecting the doer with the tremendous force for good in the universe. As a person exists more and more in oneness with cosmic love, the good he or she can do increases exponentially, for everyone is teaching others by who he is and who he is becoming. (105)

Every being in every Universe has two requirements: continuous learning and service to others. The idea of performing some kind of service often seems impossible to people because their lives are so busy as it is. But then people discover that their realities change once they have survived a natural disaster or suffered a serious illness or been through a near-death experience. They arrive at the realization that all are one; when one person has a problem, it affects everyone. Survivors learn to make time in their routines to do something extra for others.... A person's first criterion in deciding what kind of service to perform should be to do something in a field he loves. There must be passion. (105-106)

[human beings as light]

People in service are called Lightworkers because their appearance is becoming brighter and brighter. One of the ways a person can become aware of his own brightness is to pay attention on a visit to a crowded supermarket, department store, or any place where there are lots of children. They stare at people whose Light is unusually bright.

At those times when life is flowing well and a person is feeling harmony and expansive, the atoms of the body are able to absorb increasingly more Light. Eventually, the body's cells reach critical mass of Light containment....

The Source, the Creator, God — all are names for Divine Love Energy that expresses Itself in Light. It is time for people to reprogram their thinking to accept that the walls, chairs and floors that are everywhere and that seem so dense are made up of that same divine energy and therefore, are made of Light. Thought alone has densified them.... It is possible to imagine the molecular structure of everything as vibrating faster and containing more space and to visualize the material world as loving, moving energy and particles of Light. (106-107)

release and go with the flow

People would do well to relax and enjoy life. It is time to allow... people to solve their own problems.... Others cannot learn their lessons unless there is an absence of interference.... Now is the time when people need to distance themselves from getting caught up in solving other people's problems....

Eighty percent of people's dilemmas would immediately disappear if they could forget all references to the past.... What a person did at another time, how he reacted last week or even fifty years ago was the best way he knew to act at the time. No one is to blame. Everyone is to be forgiven. Each person is attracting all the experience he needs for the lessons he has wanted to learn. Everyone in a person's life mirrors the feelings that person has for himself.... It is very natural to have periods of doubt, and no one is immune to that. [But i]nstead of berating themselves, it would be better if they were to ask their guides for help, eat a hot fudge sundae, sit in a bubble bath or take the afternoon off to enjoy something they have wanted to do for a long time. (109-110)

past lives: pressures and processing

It is important to learn simply to trust the process....

People must believe deep in their hearts that they have chosen to be here at this particular time to share the most exciting event in Earth's history....

...Some people have come back from the future to help Earth birth herself into the fifth dimension. Many of them will be teachers and healers of the future. Now they are the disseminators of truth, and they will take the seeds of wisdom with them whereever they go. Some people might not work with this information for months or years, some will begin to change their lives tomorrow. It doesn't matter. Each one is on his or her own schedule. (111-112)

personal integration

... When all thinking is consciously under the direction of the higher self, a person quickly evolves.... Everyone is becoming a Creator.

As all three areas — physical/etheric, emotional and mental — come into harmony, people will no longer be negatively affected by anything or anyone.... Personal growth will keep pace with planetary growth. Each person will shine forth to all humanity, not alone but connected, Light to Light, with all others at his or her vibrational frequency (115-116).

In summary, it is time to start letting go of [our attachment to] the material world.... It is also vital for a person to [know that] he is creating his reality, moment by moment. Trusting in the perfect timing of all events and desires in life is essential, as is learning to recognize synchronistic events and take advantage of them.

Humans must learn to have patience with themselves and love the bodies they have chosen... (116).

Sacred Choices

how humans relate to earth

...[A] mistake people make is that they want to change the planet. They want to stop deforestation, stop the pollution affecting the atmosphere and the water supplies, and stop inhumane treatment of animals, along with many other issues. They argue among themselves in their various groups about the best way to accomplish these goals. What they have forgotten is that Earthly perfection can be patterned only upon individual perfection, and to arrive at human perfection, it is necessary to look at the self as an organism similar to the planet.

Earth's oceans, rivers and streams correspond to the emotional body of the human being. That means emotions affect everything in the body that is fluid, especially the glands and lymphatic system. Negative emotions are highly contagious. As a person evolves, he or she becomes more focused, and eventually, the power of a single individual's negative emotions could kill someone. It has been said that two minutes of anger poison the human system for up to nine months. Anger produces a chemical that compromises the immune system, and it creates sediment that clogs the normal flow of emotions. Feelings of resentment are said to be a common factor in cancer patients. Scientists have now isolated a chemical produced by laughter which is being administered to cancer patients at $40,000 per treatment. Negative emotions also cause confusion and distortion of incoming information, while positive emotion promote healing and inner peace....

The physical land masses of Earth relate to the physical body. As long as a person's body is ill or in pain, that sensation will be carried into the Earth Mother. The diseased bodies of those who died of illness and are buried in the ground continue to negatively affect Earth. Some of the poisons ingested by humans are from crop pesticides which also contaminate the soil. So it is clear that the problem is circular....

The atmosphere of Earth relates to the mental body.... Scientific tests have revealed how much of the body's energy is expended through thought, and it was learned that worry uses up energy reserves much more quickly than any other kind of thought. It is far better to focus on uplifting words such as beauty, joy, peace, harmony, angels and love. (121-122, 125)

humans are spirits with bodies

It is extremely important now that all humans consciously remember that they are spirits that have bodies. Never speak of those bodies in any way that is less than positive. It is vital to remember than the brain believes everything its owner says or thinks and it then creates that reality.

People can no longer afford to gossip or speak negatively of others. What they do not like about others is always a reflection of what they do not like about themselves....

...It is good to speak the truth but also to realize that truth is little more than an opinion on the third-dimensional plane.... Truths are pictures drawn in the mind; [and] it is wise to keep that mind open, yet discerning...

...It is important to take in the information that resonates personally and either discard the rest or, preferably, put it on a mental shelf until later; many concepts must await their proper moment. (124-125)

Appendix D

lessons of love

At this time, all of life is about learning the lessons of love.... These critical lessons include taking responsibility, identifying what is of value in life and understanding that there are no victims and no accidents.... People give themselves one test after another until they are sure they have mastered a given situation. Everyone chooses to be in the right place at the right time with exactly the right people who will help them learn a particular lesson.

Everything is either love or a lesson in love. (125)

humans as creators

It is imperative that people understand their lives moment by moment. They should be making it as loving and perfect and protected as they can imagine to be. The more people become convinced that their divine selves are their true selves, the more they move into perfection. At that point it is no longer necessary for them to surround themselves with white Light, for they are Light! The higher their vibration, the more Light they reflect outward (126).

... Each person must learn to see perfection in everything — and so it will be. People are rising into higher vibrations as each day passes. As they grow in perfection — not only their own perfection but the perfection they see in others — that energy is directly reflected into the planet. That will create the millennium all are longing for. Peace in the heart creates peace on Earth (128).

[ascension for earth and humanity]

The Great Spiritual Being who ensouls the Earth Mother is shedding her dense shell with all its imperfections. In its place will be a most radiant mantle of Light emanations. Her new grid lines are already blazing with crystalline energy as she aligns with a new pole star. Earth will stabilize once again. The rays of all the guiding planets will flow directly into each area of the world, as required. A bubble of Christed energy will slowly create a new atmosphere and under that sparkling canopy there will be no violent storms, no wrathful winds or devastating earthquakes. Everything within the loving embrace of Mother Earth will be tenderly and lovingly cared for.

Magnificent etheric geometric Cities of Light will once again radiate their brilliance. Many will be constructed with walls made from rays of Light. The process of building them will entail cooperation with the living intelligence of the elements. Structures can then be fashioned by thought. Translucent temples will again shine in the sun and be used as they were originally intended. One of the purposes will be to communicate with the Higher Intelligences.

Gold will be recognized for its beauty as ornamentation, never again to be used financially. Nothing will be owned. Everything will be shared for the benefit of all. There will be no need for doors or locks and keys; hearts and homes will be open. Even Earth herself will be open.

She will be one of the most frequently visited sites in the universe. Travel will be easier then because Earth is moving from her position at the distant edge of the galaxy to a new location much closer to the Great Central Sun as a direct result of her greatly intensified vibration. Earth will be recognized for the successful experiment in duality and density that has led her to unparalleled splendor....

Humans will move on to future realities but will long to return from time to time. All the universe will continue to value the experimentation that was carried out on the radiant little blue planet at the edge of the galaxy. In spite of the many beings which make up each human, the beings that are here now have played the most unique and invaluable role in helping to free Mother Earth from the third dimension and birth into the fifth dimension. These special individuals will always be remembered with deepest respect from those existing in every dimension.

All the angels from the Heavenly realms that surround and penetrate Earth salute humans with their music of the spheres and send their loving appreciation.

    Joy!

        Love!

            Namaste! (128-130)

Appendix D

author endnotes

chapter 5

[1] Pranic breathing utilizes Chi, Qi or universal energy in yoga-style breathing.

[2] Holotropic Breathwork is a method or approach to self-exploration originated by Stanislav Grof, M.D.

Appendix E: Excerpts from <u>Return of the Children of Light</u>[1]

Sacred geometry applies at so many different levels.[2] We find it in our physical anatomies[3] and in the architecture of our cathedrals and other sacred structures. We find it linking sacred sites and cast across the surface of our planet like a series of tuning forks, we find it in the energetic template cradling our planet in a net or grid-like weave, and interplanetarily and intergalactically we find it in the choreography of relationship danced between specified planetary and galactic chakras. Polich paints for us here a sequential history dating back to Lemurian and Atlantean times of galactic efforts to seed our planet with divine consciousness. She touches on sacred sites and sacred geometries as tuning forks[4] of sorts, offers an informative account of similarities in the Incan, Andean, and Mayan prophecies, and subsequently comforts us with her interpretative scenarios of these prophecies unfolding. She is gentle in her overview and does not evoke greater fear or uncertainty in these already challenging times preceding the closing of the Mayan calendar.[5] She sketches for us dreams of collective transformation and futures of unity, wholeness, and both/ands, all joyfully beyond the three-dimensionality of polarity, dualities, and either/ors.

---

[1] Please see *Sources Cited* under Polich.

[2] Please see Page 123-130.

[3] Please see *addendum* to this introduction in *Appendix E*.

[4] Credited to Sig Lowgren, Polich 111.

[5] The date given for this event is usually positioned around the December solstice of 2012.

addendum to the introduction to appendix e

Christine Page, M.D., in her brilliant work on Spiritual Alchemy, suggests that in order to heal the rifts around our planet, indeed, in order to resolve these differences, we must come in a spirit of peace and unity without baggage and without the usual prespecifications that are little more than our defenses against losing control. She further suggests that there is no longer an optional theatre for the qualities of love and unity — just one of necessity. However, in order to have this ability to address the rifts that punctuate our planet, we need first as individuals to heal our personal rifts and woundedness — that is, our own inner rifts and woundedness. She associates areas of planetary strife, like Iraq, South Africa, Turkey, Tibet, Central America, New York and California, with rifts in the Earth's core mirrored by echoing tears in the ethers above, which then produce those portals or easy access points to the multidimensional. These portals are the sites of fought-over power already known for thousands of years, although less readily known or expressed on the contemporary scene.

An ancient manner of drawing opposing sides together in love and unity is through the creation of the sacred shape called the vesica piscis.[6] This shape is created by passing the circumference of one circle through the center point of another circle. The resulting "fish-shaped doorway" (Page 144) is the "entry point into interdimensional awareness, unity, ecstasy, and Christ Consciousness which . . . evokes the soul's connection with its Source" (Page 144).[7] Let me back up slightly to indicate that this Universal Consciousness — this Christed Consciousness — certainly extends over a far broader period than the two-thousand years since Jesus the Christed one's human birthdate. Let me also suggest that the vesica piscis ellipse is thought by Page (145) and others to express the gist of the familiar line from scripture: "For when two or more are gathered . . . there I am in the midst of them." (St. Matthew ch. 18 v20). And it is credited with being that remarkable quintessential place of "unconditional potentiality" (Page, *Level 1 Seminar*). Many believe that psychological and psycho-spiritual consultations and any number of psychic guidance

Vesica Piscis [6]

---

[6] Page, Spiritual Alchemy 144.

[7] Robert Lawlor, in his hugely respected work on Sacred Geometry, suggests that few geometric shapes are invested with the range of meaning suffusing the vesica (Lawlor 33). His verbal sketch as follows is certainly convincing:

"The overlapping circles – an excellent representation of a cell, or any unity in the midst of becoming dual – form a fish-shaped central area which is one source of the symbolic reference to Christ as a fish. Christ, as a universal function, is symbolically this region which joins together heaven and earth, above and below, creator and creation.

The fish is also the symbolic designation of the Piscean Age, and consequently the Vesica is the dominant geometric figure for this period of cosmic and human evolution, and is the major thematic source for the cosmic temples of this age in the west, the Gothic cathedrals.

Jesus as the centre of the Vesica carries the idea of the non-substantial, universal 'Christic' principle entering into the manifest world of duality and form. The Piscean Age has been characterized as that of the formal embodiment of spirit, manifesting a deeper penetration of spirit into form, with a concurrent deepening of the materialization of spirit: the Word becomes flesh." (Lawlor 33-35)

modalities (tarot, spirit releasement therapy, soul re-creation therapy, integrated energy therapy, reiki, jyorei, and other subtle and physical energy therapies) could all be better served by first positioning themselves within a vesica piscis ellipse. It appears that within such a space people don't experience the fear of getting lost and they even seem to welcome being in it. Also, the process of whatever modality is chosen is markedly accelerated. The vesica piscis serves as a shape of initiation, a doorway between one place and another, or from one dimension into another (Page, *Level 1 Seminar*).

Returning to our personal healing of interior rifts, we are blessed with many examples of this sacred vesica piscis elliptical geometry in the human anatomy:

The vulva of the female form is that sacred place wherefrom the body form chosen by the newly reincarnating soul moves from the safety of the collective connection into that realm of spiritual amnesia through which he or she blesses him or herself in the development of that self-consciousness that learns ultimately to reconnect with the consciousness of the collectivity.

The "gap in the diaphragm" (Page 145) is another sacred place through which in physical terms the major blood vessels and the esophagus pass from the chest to the abdomen. Symbolically that sacred place represents our passage from the three lower personal chakras to the transpersonal ones above.

The vocal chords next draw our attention as we move up our anatomy pointing out the vesica piscis geometries. They represent the shift from living out the dictées of our personal will to living in harmony *with* and at the direction *of* Divine Will.

And finally, our eyes, which represent "the transition from a world of structure to one of pure light where our inner and outer worlds become a true reflection of each other and allow us to know our soul without distraction, attachment or bias" (Page 147).

Vesica piscis geometry appears also in sacred structures. The naves of many churches and cathedrals were created on the ratio of one to the square root of three, which is the precise ratio established between the sides of a rectangle placed around a vesica piscis ellipse. Furthermore, the use of this sacred geometry would indicate that the designers of these structures intended precisely for them to serve by helping humanity attune itself through toning in harmony with the frequency of the given structure for the purpose of reaching a level of vibration harmonious with Source — indeed in perfect union or communion with Source (Page 147).

Another way of bringing this sacred attunement quality of the vesica piscis energy into our lives and the healing of our interior rifts and into the raising of our consciousness and our interior frequency to one of love and unity, is through meditation. It is suggested that one sits facing a friend or a partner to do this work, or one can place an empty chair opposite one to hold the space for that invited Spirit being or guide or for that aspect of one's consciousness or one's anatomy that one desires to know more well or in whose overview wisdom one desires to share.

addendum to Appendix E

Dr. Page's meditation guidance is as follows:

> Sit comfortably, close your eyes and, with the help of breath, allow the body to start to relax. As you sink deeper into the chair or wherever you are sitting, continue to release any tension in the body using the breath.
>
> As the muscles ease, on the out-breath let go of thoughts of the past and then the thoughts of the future, bringing your mind gently to the present, relaxed and focused only on the breath. Now take your awareness inside, conscious of the movement of the chest and perhaps the heart beating but only as a passing observation. And go deeper.
>
> Move your awareness to the core of your being without effort or hurry and go deeper. From that place, take your awareness to the area of the heart chakra, the center of the chest and bring to mind a time when you have felt your heart open with feelings of joy, happiness and love. Perhaps it was with your grandchildren or with your partner or when watching a beautiful sunset or when your dog came to greet you. Whatever the experience, expand the feelings in the heart by adding color, sounds, aromas and touch and smile to yourself as the memory expands to include other people or a deepening of the connection.
>
> Now imagine your heart is like a vessel or chalice, filling with joy and happiness from the experience. Watch and feel as it becomes full and the happiness starts to spread out first to your physical body (and especially to areas of disharmony or pain) and then to the subtle bodies. No effort, no forcing, just allowing as the love and joy radiates out from your heart. If the feeling starts to decrease, simply return to the memory and using visual, auditory or kinesthetic aids, fill the heart again.
>
> Now the energy is radiating out beyond your body and in all directions around you, no effort. In particular, the joy spreads out towards your partner or towards the part of you with which you wish to engage. Simply allow the energy to flow without "sending" or trying, merging your joy with that of your partner or whoever sits opposite. Be conscious of their presence as your circles meet, observe the feeling without analysis. Let the joy continue to flow and allow yourself to bathe in the state of bliss, unity and peace that develops. If you can hold the memory with your eyes open, gently open your eyes and see how the flow may change when eye contact is added.
>
> From this place, healing takes place naturally, although we can send out a specific intention on a wave of joy. It's also a wonderful place from which to communicate with someone where trust may have been an issue or when you wish to reach a deeper level of communion. If you are working with a part of yourself, you can ask this part questions and wait for answers directly into your heart without the need for words.
>
> When you are complete, simply give silent thanks and slowly draw the energies back into your body and your heart, knowing that you have been enriched by the exchange and this place always awaits you. (Page 148-149)

appendix e[8]

[concluding the Mayan calendar]

It is no coincidence that the Mayan calendar ends in 2012 on December 21, the winter solstice. The current world-age... is waning. The 5,125-year period that began in 3112 B.C. and marks the current cycle of seedings is drawing to a close. The Maya predict that this cycle of time... will end in great earthquakes—a notion that could be a metaphor for great cultural changes. However, it is important to remember that the simultaneous conjunction of the solstice sun with the galactic center offers a potential for great spiritual transformation and rebirth.

In this context, it is noteworthy that a very rare planetary alignment will occur on December 24, 2011, one year before the Mayan calendar ends. On that date all the planets in our solar system will be spaced 30 degrees apart. Statistically, this phenomenon could only occur once every 45,200 years.$_2$ Apparently, the Maya foresaw this alignment and thus, to them, the year 2012 was far more than the end of a precessional cycle; it was a major galactic event.

Everywhere there are signs of **pachacuti**;[9] great planetary changes are now abundant. Global weather patterns have become erratic, resulting in massive droughts, famines, hurricanes, and earthquakes. In addition, rain forests are burning at increasing rates, and the number of species on the planet is rapidly dwindling. Suggested causes include global warming, the depletion of the ozone layer, El Niño, La Niña, nuclear testing, sun spot activity, and the encroachment of technological civilization. Whatever the cause, it is clear our planet is undergoing massive changes. Even so, **pachacuti** is likely to be a cultural, perceptual shift rather than a physical event. (94-95)

understanding light dynamics

God-seeds act with focused, conscious intent. They understand light dynamics, realizing that each thought and each emotion they experience sets light in motion. They take responsibility for the light that flows through them, aware that they have chosen to bring this light to Earth.

As god-seeds mature, they become more and more luminous, eventually becoming illuminated ones. They develop the ability to pull in higher frequencies of light and to radiate these into the world. They heal, teach, and serve where needed, making their light available to individuals and to world situations that can benefit from healing. They understand that they are merely servants of the light, here to assist the planet and its inhabitants in achieving and maintaining a higher level of functioning.

God-seeds comprehend the fundamental truth that has been verified by quantum physics—that light is responsive to intent. Quantum physics has shown that the nature of light as we perceive it depends solely on the intention of the perceiver,

---

[8] Please see *Sources Cited* under Polich.

[9] *Pachacuti* translates as "a time of great physical or psychological transformation" (Polich 138).

since whether light takes the form of a wave or a particle depends on the intent of the observer. The same rules apply to inner light, whose form of manifestation depends on the intent of the human shaping it. We need to be fully conscious of how we use our intent. This is what it means to be awake.

The conscious use of intent is the key to the next leap in human evolution. To grasp the meaning of this, we need to realize that our true human potential has not yet been developed due to the devastating consequences of our individual and collective false perceptions. We must act knowing that our intentions create the world, rather than feeling like we are being acted upon by outside forces beyond our control.

Because matter is light frozen in form, we have within us the wavelike nature of pure light. The new physics tells us that at a subatomic level the physical vehicle that forms our body looks, feels, and acts like physical light, The light that informs our consciousness is nonphysical light. Both aspects of the light that fills our being have distinct internal orders, but they are governed by a higer order that may not be limited by the physical laws of this space/time. The human hologram is therefore a dynamic form capable of endless expansion.

We have been brought up to believe many false concepts about ourselves, some of which come from Newtonian physics and the Cartesian worldview. There is nothing inherently wrong with these systems of thought; they have just been overapplied. They cannot describe all aspects of reality. Many other falsehoods we live with come from our conventional religious systems. For example, the Judeo-Christian tradition gives us the story of the Garden of Eden, a myth that unfortunately has been misinterpreted and causes great harm to our collective psyche. It is possible we were never banished from the garden, and we did not sin. Thus, we are not unworthy spiritually.

How human experience came into existence can also be explained in terms of light descending deeper into matter and becoming frozen in form—the natural process of involution that preceded the evolutionary period that is now approaching. This was a necessary phase of the process of light interpenetrating the denser realms of the physical aspect of creation. Creation, in this context, did not end in 6 days, but is an ongoing process. We are being created "into the form and similitude of God" right now.

With the advent of higher consciousness, the light that has been hidden in form is awakening to its potential. We are now shifting from a frozen involutionary process into a dynamic evolutionary process. As human god-seeds, our light is rising upward just as the sprout rises and reaches to the light. As we reach upward, we pull ourselves from the lower frequency of matter to higher, more refined realms. As we become fully conscious, we will raise all matter to a higher frequency, literally infusing all matter with higher vibrations of light.

This is why we are here and why light entered matter. There never has been any separation. The ancient people of Mesoamerica and Peru knew who they were, believing that their ancestors came from the stars and that they were children of the light. We forgot who we are, falling asleep in the dark and potent realms of matter. Now ... we are beginning to collectively awaken. The children of light are returning. (106-107)

In veiled language, esoteric teachings tell us that the divine aspect of the human form came from the stars and that the cluster of the Pleiades provided the blueprints for human consciousness. These blueprints may be thought of as actual codes of light that have been implanted within the human form.[9] These light codes can be seen as divine thought forms that provide the catalysts that awaken in mankind the light that brings higher consciousness.

A helpful analogy for this human process is the seed of any common plant. For example, the seed of any flower has within it a hidden code contained in the plant's DNA that becomes activated under certain conditions: time of year, amount of sunlight and moisture. The code causes the seed to sprout, grow, flower, bear fruit, produce seed, and then repeat the same cycle. Similarly, the light codes within the human form may be viewed as spiritual DNA, as the inner forces that trigger the process of enlightenment. The ultimate maturation of the god-seed in each human being is divinity, an example of which is Christ consciousness....

According to some esoteric accounts, such as Hurtak's and Sumerian and Babylonian creation myths from which later Hebraic creation myths may have derived, a purpose of the spiritual human, the seed, was to create a new species capable of carrying the light of higher consciousness.[13] This species is known as the Adamic Race, or the Adam Kadmon. Gnostic and other texts emphasize that the Adam Kadmon is a continually evolving species of light made in "the image and similitude" of the Elohim (angels)....

Many of these traditions tell of androgynous god-like beings known in early Hebraic accounts as the Elohim. Within the hierarchy of the spiritual world, the Elohim are considered mighty angels who embody high intelligence and creative powers, and who sit at the right hand of God himself. (29-31)

Andean teacher Juan Nuñez del Prado helps his students learn to distinguish between heavy, dense energies and refined energies. When we express negative emotions such as fear, hate, and anger, we are involved with dense energies and lower frequency currents. By contrast, when we express more positive emotions like love and kindness, we are dealing with more refined energies and higher frequency currents. The lower the frequency, the less consciousness and light; the higher the frequency, the more consciousness and light. It makes perfect sense that as we express more of our true divine natures, the energy we create is more refined.

In our universe all physical light is a reflection of nonphysical light originating from pure consciousness that preceded and gave rise to form. Thus, although we exist in the physical form, we are a reflection of the divine light of a higher order. Because the ancients understood the potency of divine reflection and that the light of consciousness is not limited to the laws of the physical universe, their ceremonial sites were built to reflect both inner light and divine consciousness.

Gary Zukav believes that we are evolving from one frequency spectrum to another. As humans we perceive a specific color spectrum and our five basic senses function within a limited range; yet we also know invisible rays of light border the limited spectrum we see, and that higher and lower frequencies of light exist than we can perceive with the five senses. Nonphysical light also has a frequency range. We exist at a certain level of consciousness, a certain frequency of light, but we may now be making a jump to a higher frequency spectrum of light—light far more refined.

We often associate more refined energies and light qualities with spiritually evolved beings, such as great world teachers like Jesus and Mohammed. They represent the fully empowered human seed whose role is to show us what we will become.

However, to many, this potential has seemed unattainable on Earth. It is critical at this point in the evolution of our collective human consciousness that we understand that it is not unattainable and come forward to claim our true identity and divine potential. The god-seed in each one of us is already invested with divine energy, the same potential that was realized by mythical god-men of the past.

The awakening process requires that we begin to function as beings of light. As Zukav reminds us, we are dynamic beings of light capable of regulating the energy that flows through our systems with our thoughts and intents:

> The Light that flows through your system is Universal energy. It is the Light of the Universe. You give that Light form. What you feel, what you think, how you behave, what you value and how you live your life reflect the way you are shaping the light that is flowing through you. They are thought forms, the feeling forms and the outer forms that you have given to Light. They reflect the configuration of your personality, your space-time being.[15]

When you become integrated with the light that flows through your system, as Zukav says, you become like laser light, coherent, a beam of light in which every wave precisely reinforces every other wave. The integrated human, the god-seed, is being a laser of light. (104-105)

[sacred sites]

There are many tools available to help the human god-seed awaken, and sacred sites around the world are some of the most powerful....

There are sacred sites all over the world. Stonehenge, Mecca, Iona, Haleakala, the Ganges, Delphi, Palenque, Jerusalem, the Egyptian pyramids, Chartres, Chaco Canyon, Teotihuacán, and Machu Picchu are but a few, and people are visiting such sites in astonishing numbers....

There is no question that individuals can ... charge physical space with higher vibrational energy, and that sacred sites are profoundly spiritual places. However, there are also unique physical characteristics associated with sacred sites. Many of the sacred sites on this planet are thought to be connected by an almost invisible grid of astronomical and geometrical lines. Russian scientists have found evidence of a faint pattern of magnetic lines running around our planet that make the shape of a dodecahedron (a 12-sided figure) imposed on an icosahedron (a 20-sided figure).[3] It has been speculated by some researchers that this is evidence that the planet was once a large crystal or that it was energized in some manner by a crystalline core.[4] Scientists studying this phenomenon have found that the locations of the most ancient civilizations and their sacred sites occur along the magnetic lines of this planetary icosahedron.[5]

Meteorological and geological maps have established that maximal and minimal atmospheric pressure areas are found precisely at the nodes of the dodecahedron. These nodes are the areas where hurricanes originate and where the oceans have huge vortices of current. Core faults as well as unusual features like the Bermuda Triangle also occur on the nodes.[6] Rudolf Steiner, the founder of a field of study called anthroposophy, has said that as a living entity, Earth would energetically take the form of a dodecahedron-icosahedron,[7] a statement that correlates with the findings of Buckminster Fuller.[8] Another Russian, Vitaly Kabachenko, who studied maps of the Earth taken from outer space, found that they showed a grid barely noticeable as black streaks on the ocean floor and in the sky.[9] Others, including Aimé Michel, a French writer who has written about the UFO phenomenon, have said that UFO sitings tend to occur along similar magnetic lines that also form a planetary grid.[10] Moreover, increasing numbers of people believe that Earth is a living organism and that its body is intersected with *ley* (energy) lines that function just like the acupuncture meridians found in the human body. It may be appropriate to think of such a grid as the energy body of the earth.

There has been much speculation about the origins of such grids. After reviewing evidence found on many ancient maps, geomancer and author John Michell concluded that in our prehistory someone, or some group, precisely mapped the entire globe and laid out a network of astronomical and geometrical lines that cross the entire planet. According to Michell, many of the most sacred sites are found on these lines, including sites made of vast blocks of stone that function as massive astrological instruments. He has concluded that the human predecessors who built these sites had to have had advanced technologies and "remarkable powers."[11]

Not surprisingly, Teotihuacán and many of the other ancient sites of Mesoamerica and Peru are found along these grids. Apparently, based upon their experiences, the ancients of these regions and elsewhere believed that the planetary energy lines had powers related to healing and the expansion of consciousness. (109-111)

aspects of sacred space

There are numerous theories regarding sacred space. Sig Lowgren, a dowser who has studied many sacred sites around the world, believes that most of these sacred sites were located and designed to enhance contact with spiritual realms. He has suggested that through the use of sacred geometry a physical space that has the right characteristics could actually be tuned like a musical instrument so it could resonate at a specific frequency. After dowsing a number of sacred sites, he has found that most of them are places where yin and yang energies within the earth converge. The yin, feminine-receptive energy, is found where there are domes and veins of underground water, while the yang, or masculine force, is carried by straight beams of energy or *ley* lines.[12]

We know that certain people (dowsers) have the ability to sense underground water and magnetic and telluric forces.... Subsequent research has shown that the magnetic sensors in the human body are located in the pineal gland,[13] which implies that theoretically, everyone has the ability to sense such currents.

Lowgren has found that the energies measurable at sacred sites vary throughout the calendar year. We know that many of our ancient sites were designed for use on solstices, equinoxes, and other specific dates....

Lowgren also discovered that when an energy *ley* line aligns with the rising and setting of the sun, the *ley* line actually becomes more potent....

Ritual sites also employ sacred geometry—the geometry found in nature and consisting of the sets of correspondences, geometrically expressed by ratios.... It is the geometry found in the formation of matter at the subatomic level, in the natural motions of astronomical phenomena of the universe, and in organic forms of plant life. In brief, sacred geometry shows us the blueprint of all creation.

Encoded into many sites are the sacred geometric ratios of creation, which reflect the ancient law of correspondence—as above, so below....

In addition, there are other aspects of correspondence that may be relevant to sacred sites, such as the principle of harmonic resonance. When two objects resonate in a harmonic state, energy is exchanged between them, which may be relevant to the energy dynamics that exist at some of the sacred places on our planet. Correspondence can be a function of form, as in sacred geometry; it can also be a function of vibration, as in harmonic resonance.

Research done at sacred sites has also shown that the sites themselves often contain unusual amounts of natural radioactivity and magnetic anomalies. (111-113)

The sacred sites of our world share one fundamental characteristic—they are all places where spirit communicates. For some that communication takes the form of heightened awareness, while others experience archetypal imagery or altered states—all encounters with the divine.

Virtually all of the ceremonial centers in Mesoamerica and Peru—including Teotihuacán, Machu Pichu, Palenque, and Monte Albán—were built for the express purpose of divine communication although we do not know the specifics of how these sites were used or their purpose in a larger world context. Perhaps, as John Michell suggests, they are part of a larger complex of structures that ring the planet, a type of tuning fork that was deliberately built by divine beings, or perhaps arose independently from a collective impulse....

Many of the ruins of antiquity like the Great Pyramid and Stonehenge were designed as astronomical and geodetic markers that theoretically aligned our world with the greater cosmic whole. (113)

doorways of harmonic frequency

There is no doubt that the heightened energy experienced at such sites is perceptible and tangible. It vibrates through our chakra systems and energy bodies. Although the stones that make up such sites appear to be visibly solid, we know that they are energy fields and that all matter has frequency—at least at the subatomic level. We now know that at a subatomic level what we perceive of as matter may simply be bands of vibration bound within a field, and that although most of these frequencies are too minimal for us to measure, they are not necessarily too small for us to perceive. (115)

sacred sites and altered states

Dragon Project[10] director Paul Devereux suggests that sacred sites were not intended to be used in a normal state of *consciousness but in altered states, which can be induced in many ways, such as through drumming, ritual, prayer, and dreaming, as well as mind-altering drugs.$_{22}$ Moreover, the energy fields of the sites themselves often promote such altered states or perceptual shifts.... It is entirely possible that the codings imprinted in sacred sites automatically shift the assemblage points of people at the site (116-118).*

understanding sacred correspondence

We know that the people of Mesoamerica and Peru built and used sacred sites primarily for ceremonial purposes. As we have seen, there is substantial evidence that they were built to awaken higher states of consciousness and to create opportunities for divine communication. After flourishing, the ceremonial areas of these regions were abandoned. Prior to abandoning these sites, it is likely that our predecessors deliberately sealed certain critical features of the sites energetically as a form of protection. Since they knew a time of darkness was coming, they may have realized that as the human god-seed descended further into the world of matter, it would lose the ability to function in the higher dimensions, and thus they locked the portals with these sacred libraries of divine consciousness. They probably knew that the power hidden within the sacred sites themselves would help to catalyze the future awakening of the seed.

There is a simple but ancient formula for accessing this hidden power, a key well known by the builders—the law of sacred correspondence, the principle of "as above, so below." Basically, the power of these sites can be accessed at any time when the light that shines from below is equal to the light that shines from above. In our space/time, this means that to access this power our own personal light must reflect the higher light, our frequency must resonate with a higher harmonic, thus assuring that access to such power is never given to those who are spiritually unprepared.

In this context, it is important to remember that all living things emit light.... Eastern teachings tell us that the living light is encoded in our form. The ancient concept of the macrocosm as microcosm also tells us that the greater divine life (light) is reflected in the human body. Expressed in another manner, this means that the Adam Kadmon, the spiritual human created "in the image and likeness" of the Elohim, has encoded within it a divine blueprint. Through knowledge of the science of vibration, we can learn to unlock these mysteries. This is how the Adam Kadmon (the light body) unfolds from the implicate order. (118-119)

the elevation of collective consciousness

We are approaching an unprecedented time in the development of human consciousness when the sixth sun will catalyze a new human evolution. Never has it been more important for us to awaken to our cosmic origins. We desperately need to break out of the box that limits our perception of our potential. Our narrow attitudes, sensory limitations, fears of the unknown, and forgetfulness have trapped us for far too long. Fortunately, the libraries of antiquity left to us by our forebears

---

[10] A project developed to study the energies at sacred sites.

offer us a way to remember who we are. When we approach these libraries with receptivity and in a spirit of gratitude, they will reveal their secrets.

As we have discussed, it is possible that ancient ceremonial sites were part of a giant grid of energy that surrounds the planet....

...José Argüelles tells us we are now in the time of the great synchronization that will result in the quickening and transformation of matter....

Moreover, he believes that various releases of nuclear energy since 1945 have affected the vibratory structure of Earth itself. To compensate for this vibrational shift, he predicts that the crystalline core of Earth will make an adjustment in the form of a series of waves until a new level of harmonic resonance is reached, resulting in a vibratory shift in the planetary light body itself.[30] Argüelles explains that this is our galactic destiny, part of the development of a fully conscious planetary light body.

> Here is the picture of what has been happening. Slowly, over the eons, at Earth's core, the iron crystal lodestone of her [the Earth's] harmonic gyroscope has been emitting the resonant frequencies that keep her in orbit. These resonant frequencies have a particular shape or form, for form follows frequency. This is why Plato described the Earth as being like a leather ball sewn together from twelve different pieces, creating a dodecahedron or twelve interfaced pentagons. The vertices between the pentagonal pieces define the structure of the resonate body of the Earth as the frequency emissions reach the surface.
>
> As the core resonance continuously emanates out to the surface of the Earth and beyond, an etheric grid comes into being, forming the foundations of the planetary light body. Attuned through the frequency patterns of the DNA infrastructure, animal migration patterns and human settlements tend to conform to the lines and nodal points of the grid. Of course, the grid is warped and reshaped by tectonic plate activity, variable shifts in terrain and atmosphere, and solar-galactic triggered fluctuations in the electromagnetic field of the planet itself. Nonetheless, anchored at the poles, amplified at times by (to us) unforeseen and imperceptible shifts in the galactic program, the continuous pulsation of the grid slowly shapes the infrastructure of the planetary light body.[31]...

What this may look like from the human perspective is a gradual shift in consciousness to an understanding of a new worldview. This new worldview will make it evident that the world we live in is a living entity, and that it is part of a larger whole. We will be able to perceive that all matter is energy, that we are wave-like, that we are in constant communication with the whole. Through this shift in consciousness, we will begin to function as multi-dimensional beings, and we will realize we have potentials beyond anything yet dreamed of, adding our heightened light vibration to the Earth's own.

As these new human potentials begin to unfold we will fully grasp that we are indeed god-seeds. As god-seeds we have the power of conscious intent. We can learn to bring potential into form. Our DNA is specially programmed, encoded with light-sensitive patterns that will unfold the new humans we are evolving into. This new human is a being of light, capable of functioning with a fully activated light body.

In order to unlock the potentials in our DNA, we need to start perceiving ourselves as beings of light and understand how to use conscious intent. From this viewpoint of higher consciousness, we are akin to electrons in our own molecules, which exhibit their potential when we perceive them as waves or as particles....

Many people believe that the activation of the grid, the planetary light body, is already occurring, awakening our potentials. As we individually awaken to the light within human form, the light within the planetary form is simultaneously awakening. This is occurring because within the larger whole, a new pattern is emerging—the universe is holographic....

The great and ancient ceremonial centers that ring our planet can be tools in service of the new alignment.... The new consciousness will emerge when we as a human community collectively align our vibration with the higher vibration that is awakening within the planetary light field. The doorways to divine consciousnesss, the ancient gateways, which are in actuality the next level of the implicate order, will open when "the light that comes from below is equal to the light that comes from above." (120-123)

stepping into the angel light

At some point early in the development of the universe, matter separated from light. Scientifically stated, as the universe expanded and cooled there was an uncoupling of matter and radiation. Prior to that time darkness and light were undifferentiated.[24] The first light created may have been an invisible illumination, or the light of consciousness, or the angel light.

If we look at angels in the context of recent scientific discoveries, we begin to come closer to understanding the truth of both their existence and purpose. Hildegard of Bingen, whose works were based largely on mystical awareness, wrote of angels as living light,[25] as the invisible illumination that clings to living, flying spheres,[26] and stated that angels were created to function as living mirrors of divine light....

Most classical angelologists believed there were nine hierarchies of angels. These spheres, which we can now think of as angelic fields, order all of consciousness and span from the microcosm of human existence to the macrocosm of galactic interaction....

Finding the angel light within can be an arduous process, since to do so we must let go of many limiting beliefs and entirely re-envision ourselves....

As don Miguel Ruiz tells us, to reach the angel light we have to make a perceptual shift, since the angel light is ultimately a mystical experience. And as with all mystical experiences, after we have been engendered by the light we have to come down from the mountain. When we return from a mystical experience, we find that remarkably our world has also been transformed. We see the world differently because we are different. Because we have touched the angel light, we have within us holistic vision and the other gifts of angel light. (132-133)

... The first gift of the angel light is holistic vision, the ability to see ourselves as god-seeds within an interactive galactic whole. This allows us to see who we really are and that we are all part of the light of pure consciousness. Holistic vision brings

a radical shift in perspective, not only causing us to alter self-centered and destructive patterns of behavior but also to change our thinking. In addition, holistic vision allows us to understand our inherent multi-dimensionality, enabling us to access multiple aspects of our consciousness.

In this space/time, humans have physicality, but we are more than that. We are each a part of the angel light that makes up human consciousness. And by the power of our intent, we can expand upward through the nested orders of angel light to embrace the refined light of our celestial forebears. We can do this through light that connects our consciousness to the greater whole. Like the subatomic particles that define our physical structure, we are particle-like as we participate in everyday life and wavelike as our consciousness dances in unbroken wholeness. In time it is possible to make such perceptual shifts more fluidly. Through the development of our witness consciousness (a state of detached self observation, free of judgment), we can observe ourselves shifting from one state to another and perceive our simultaneous existences as the quantum beings we truly are.

Because of our multiplicity, we can consciously move between different realms of existence. We are a particle of consciousness fixed in this space/time but also a unity of consciousness beyond time or space. The gift we receive from our multiple levels of perception is that as quantum beings we can finally understand that separation is an illusion. (133-134)

Another gift of the angel light is unconditional love. Our new holistic vision makes it clear that we exist in an unbroken wholeness that is filled with dynamic energy and is infused with intent. The intent that pervades the angel light carries one message—unconditional love. The unifying force that pulses from the formless into form, the force that rides the waves of pure light, is the force of unconditional love. Unconditional love is the vibration that comes from the central sun, the Self. It is the superluminal force that awakens the light codes hidden in the human form, which engender the human seed, creating the capacity for divine radiance.

Unconditional love is an impersonal force that will not sustain any egotistical, false sense of Self; it only sustains the light....

Unconditional love is the intent that filters from the heart of the creator and lights the hearts of the masters. It is the unifying force eternally dedicated to our awakening that filters down to this planet....

Once you grasp the nature of unconditional love you realize that there is a galactic agenda. There is a higher order of complexity that is unfolding within human consciousness as a whole. Then you receive the next gift of the angel light—humility, perhaps the hardest gift to accept. After all, we learn to function within the planetary dream because we have an ego,, and the better we function, the higher our self-importance—it is, in fact, a major obstacle. Instead, it is necessary to surrender all our false pride. (134-135)

Humility ultimately teaches us that all life is sacred—a gift of the divine union of form and the formless. The ancients ... understood that everything on the planet is sacred, including every blade of grass, flower, clump of dirt and brick. This is the critical message of the Andean masters, who perceive all objects as animate because they comprehend that everything has consciousness and acts as a receptacle of light.

When we become distracted, we slip again into perceiving things as separate, momentarily forgetting our quantum, multi-dimensional nature and losing the sacred worldview. Then as our perception shifts, we again awaken, realizing that we were seeing life from a distorted perspective. This process of reawakening is humbling and evokes deep gratitude.

The gift of gratitude leades ultimately to the practice of **ayni**. We can walk in perfect **ayni** in all worlds as the ancient ones did. As don Morales says, we can learn to perceive, think, act, and speak from a state of awareness of the sacred nature of all things. Then the world will mirror to us our sacredness. (135)

Appendix E

author endnotes

chapter 2: seedings of divine consciousness

[9] J. J. Hurtak, *The Keys of Enoch* (Los Gatos, CA: the Academy for Future Science, 1977), 54.

[11] Zecharia Stichin, *the 12th Planet* (New York: Avon Books, 1976). 336-362.

[13] See Note 9, 27-28, 54-56; See Note 11, Stichin, 336-339.

chapter 5: awakening

[2] Frank Waters, The Mexican Mystique (Athens, OH: Swallow Press, 1975), Sklower appendix, 285-304.

[15] Gary Zukav, *The Seat of the Soul* (New York: Simon and Schuster, 1989), 106.

chapter 6: libraries of antiquity

[3] Peter Tompkins, *Mysteries of the Mexican Pyramids* (New York: Harper and Row, 1976), 326.

[4] Ibid., 327.

[5] Ibid., 330-1.

[6] Ibid., 327.

[7] Ibid., 328.

[8] Ibid., 328.

[9] Ibid., 327.

[10] Ibid., 328.

[11] Ibid., 326, 328-9.

[12] Sid Lonegren, *Spiritual Dowsing* (Glastonbury: Gothic Image Publications, 1986), 34-35.

[13] Paul Devereux, *Earth Memory* (St Paul, MN: Llewllyn, 1992), 183.

[21] Michael Talbot, *The Holographic Universe* (New York: Harper Perennial, 1991), 174-6.

[22] See Note 12, 302.

[30] José Argüelles, *The Mayan Factor* (Santa Fe: Bear and Co., 1987), 147-8.

[31] Ibid., 154.

[32] See Note 21, 293.

chapter 7: stepping into the angel light

[5] Matthew Fox and Rupert Sheldrake, *The Physics of Angels* (San Francisco: Harper San Francisco, 1996). 18.

[24] See Note 5, 85.

[25] See Note 5, 138.

[26] See Note 5, 139.

Appendix F: Excerpts from Energy Blessings from the Stars[1]

Perhaps some of the information included in this appendix will seem phantasmical or even diametrically in opposition to lovingly honoured spiritual beliefs and understandings — even for persons who consider themselves supremely flexible and of an especially New Age inclination. For our mutual well-being though — yours and mine and planet Earth's and ours — please try not to let these ideas evoke strongly negative responses. Perhaps they can be allowed (accepted even) in a gently neutral style, as possible options in a present tense's ocean of multiple interpretations. Against such a tapestry of information (where the tapestry includes visions of humanity's role in the evolution of Mother Earth and of the galaxy and considerations of their possible pasts and potential futures) and cradled in its collective embrace, I can more easily address the perimeter exterior to the multi-valenced spokes that together form the sacred wheel of medicinal aromatherapy. This perimeter is not the only future path of healing, but rather an exquisite interblending of devic gifts and humanity's reception of these gifts — indeed a profound and beautiful path among other healing paths for mankind's spiritual co-evolution.

energy

IF[2]: *First let me define what I mean when I use the term "subtle energy." When we use the word "subtle" in ordinary language, it can refer to something which is difficult to detect. Similarly, I would define a subtle energy as one which cannot currently be detected by mainstream scientific instruments. The situation we're in with subtle energy is analogous to the early days of research into electricity. At that time experimenters observed that frog legs hanging from a rack would jump when the rack was hit with lightning; however, they had no understanding of electricity and no way of measuring it. We can observe*

---

[1] Please see *Sources Cited* under Essene.

[2] **IF** are the initials of one of the co-authors of Energy Blessings. His name is Irving Feurst.

effects of subtle energy, but we don't yet have standard scientific instruments for measuring and quantifying it. One day we will have such instruments and then subtle energy will be considered just as real as any other form of energy.

It appears that subtle energies, or at least many of them, don't have any mass. This makes it difficult for some people to understand how such energies can have tangible effects. However, I would like to point out that a photon (a particle of light) also has no mass. Yet bombardment by a stream of photons can produce very real effects.... Even though photons have no mass they can cause matter to move over a distance or to do "work." In a similar way, even if subtle energy has no mass, it can still do work....

... [O]ne example which illustrates both similarities and differences between physical and subtle energies is that of distant transmission. Like physical energies, subtle energies can be transmitted over large distances....

However, subtle energies appear to travel at speeds which can not be matched by physical energies. It is commonly thought that subtle energies can travel faster than light, which may seem strange to some readers. Nonetheless, a variety of explanations have been proposed by reputable scientists as to how this could happen. One of the most commonly discussed models has been proposed by William Tiller, a professor Emeritus and former head of the department of Material Sciences and Engineering at Stanford University.... Tiller's model describes electromagnetic waves as transverse waves and subtle energy waves as longitudinal waves. These subtle energy waves have been compared to pressure waves running longitudinally under the ocean. The velocities of these pressure waves are not limited by the transverse velocity of the surface waves.... What is intriguing about Tiller's model is that it can be interpreted to mean that the longitudinal subtle energy waves actually create the conventional transverse electromagnetic waves. This is in accord with the ancient spiritual wisdom that the lower vibrational planes of reality are manifested from the higher vibrational planes of reality....

... Arthur C. Clarke said that any sufficiently advanced technology looks like magic.... [However, while the use of subtle energies] may look like magic... like all subtle energy phenomenon it obeys rational principles.

... There are two other interrelated differences.... The first is that subtle energy responds much more readily to human consciousness than physical energy....

A related concept is that subtle energy can be "programmed." Readers may be familiar with programming a quartz crystal, for example. Of course, what is really being programmed is the subtle energy field associated with the crystal. (41-44)

[**IF:**] Western culture is still in its infancy in learning about subtle energy and about the energy centers already known in other cultures. For historical reasons the West learned about chakras and meridians first, and as a result, many people have assumed that this is all that there is to know, or all that is important.

We still have much to learn from these cultures with which we already have the most familiarity. For example, in Hinduism there is a vast knowledge not only of the chakras but also of the energy centers known as marmas. These are located in regions where bones, joints, muscles, ligaments, blood vessels, or nerves meet. These centers are important concentrations of life energy. As mentioned, we also have much to learn from traditions that are not as familiar to us. Sufism has knowledge about the energy centers known as lat'if, the Jewish tradition of Kabbalah has knowledge about the energy centers known as sefirot (or the Tree of Life centers), and the Hawaiian tradition of Huna knows about centers called ao. Experience has shown that combining knowledge of the chakras and meridians with work on any of these other energy centers, produces results that far exceed what can be done by working with just the chakras and meridians alone. (45-46)

[**IF:**] ... Every human being is intimately connected to Mother Earth. Indeed, the evolution of humanity as a whole and the evolution of planet Earth are inextricably intertwined. Acceleration in either evolutionary process must eventually result in an acceleration of the other; a block in either evolutionary process must eventually result in a block in the other. We can better comprehend why this is so by understanding the structure and functioning of the Earth's gridwork system.

First, let me clarify what I mean by the term "Earth's gridwork." Some people have used this term in discussing physical, electromagnetic energy. The term "Earth's gridwork" has also been used—as we use it in this book—to refer to a system of **channels** which are made up of subtle (not physical) matter and which conduct the flow of subtle (not physical) energy. A good way to understand the Earth is by analogy with a human being. A human being has a physical body and also has a nested sequence of subtle bodies, which interpenetrate and surround the physical body. Similarly, the Earth has a physical body and also has a nested sequence of subtle bodies, which interpenetrate and surround that physical Earth. The Earth's gridwork system is part of the subtle bodies of the Earth and it both interpenetrates and surrounds the physical Earth.

The energy channels which make up this system form a three dimensional matrix which is present everywhere (on land, sea, and air) and which passes through all things on the Earth, including living beings. Ley lines (which are straight lines connecting sacred sites) are sometimes, but not always, near major energy channels. The Earth's gridwork system receives, stores, transforms, and transmits subtle energy. The gridwork system has three primary functions. First, it connects all living beings to the Earth. Second, it connects all living beings to each other. Third, it receives subtle energies from humans and from spiritual beings—both beings here on Earth and non-terrestrial beings.

Sending energies to the Earth is a way that unseen spiritual beings can help humanity and at the same time fulfill their obligation to respect our free will and not be overly intrusive. These energies combine with the energies that are naturally present on our planet, both complementing them and increasing their effect.

Many people have noticed an acceleration in their personal or spiritual evolution after experiencing the energies of a sacred site, for example those at Stonehenge, England or in Sedona, Arizona, in the United States. What they are experiencing is a quicker, more concentrated form of a process which is happening to everyone on our planet simply by being in the presence of the subtle energies emitted by rocks and plants. The unseen spiritual beings who are helping humanity have been sending energies to the rocks, plants, and water of the Earth throughout history; and now that the process is shifting into a higher gear. We are receiving more energies, stronger energies, and the energies are coming in at a faster rate. This is why so many people have the feeling that our evolution is speeding up.

When we understand the interconnections made by the Earth's gridwork system, it is easier to understand the interdependence of the Earth's evolutionary process and humanity's evolutionary process. If the Earth's gridwork increases in vibrational rate or if unseen spiritual beings enrich the gridwork with a new energy, then humans and all other living beings on the Earth are positively affected. When you receive an initiation your vibrational rate goes up because your subtle bodies are enriched by the presence of a new frequency. This transformation in you spreads out through the Earth's gridwork system and will have some positive effect on her and on all the living beings which inhabit her.... Once you receive any of the initiations in this book, you will emit subtle energy frequencies which are helpful not only to yourself and others, but somewhat to Mother Earth's gridwork system and energy centers, especially her heart chakra. This will happen just by your being alive and won't require any conscious effort on your part!

    Just as a human being has seven primary chakras, so too does Mother Earth. In a way similar to the major function of our human heart chakra—which is to help harmonize, balance, and develop our other chakras—the Earth's heart chakra functions to help harmonize, balance, and develop the Earth's other chakras. The Earth's heart chakra not only works with her own chakras' energies but encourages an attitude of tolerance between different peoples, thus promoting world peace. The Earth's heart chakra is located at Shambhala, in the Northern Gobi desert. Stonehenge, which is sometimes mentioned as the Earth's heart chakra, is actually located near the Earth's hara center. In humans the hara center is located about two to three finger widths below the navel and between one to two inches inside the body; it is an important center for the distribution of energy throughout the body. Similarly the Earth's hara center is an important center for the distribution of energy throughout the Earth's subtle body gridwork system....

    ...[I]t is not even necessary for you to understand the mechanics of this process to benefit from initiation, any more than you need to understand electrical theory to benefit from turning on a light. But let me lead into our next chapter on initiation with this brief comment about the value of the energy received during this initiation process. *A subtle energy initiation results in a permanent transformation in the invisible but very real energy fields that surround and interpenetrate your physical body.* It enriches these fields by adding to them one or more frequencies of subtle energy that were not previously present. In some cases it is a higher vibrational frequency; in other cases it is simply a different frequency, thereby facilitating a qualitative change in our way of being in the world. These initiations, or energy blessings from the stars, are an exciting and valuable energy experience offered by the spiritual masters to those people interested in growth and service. (56-59)

new hope for humanity

    ... So where is all this headed? What is the future of planet Earth and of humanity? It will help us better understand the answers to these questions if we step back and look at the overall design of the universe and see how planetary and human evolution fit into that bigger picture.

    As we discussed previously, the universe is composed of two arcs of creation—the involutionary arc and the evolutionary arc. The involutionary arc is associated with the descent of spirit into matter and has been called the out-breath of God. The evolutionary arc is associate with the ascent of matter into spirit and has been called the in-breath of God. The ultimate purpose of all evolutionary processes within the universe is the integration of these two arcs, the integration of matter and spirit. At the individual level we are talking about the integration of our spiritual nature and our personality (with the personality referring to our bodies, emotions, and thoughts). Many of the problems that we humans experience are the result of different ways in which the lack of integration between our spiritual nature and our personality can manifest. Some people have an inner emptiness, even unrecognized consciously, because their personality cannot even accept the reality of the spiritual realm. Other spiritually-oriented people have great difficulty integrating their spiritual experiences and values into daily life. A number of them have difficulty even accepting their life on the physical plane and long to return to higher realms.

There is certainly meant to be a natural polarity or tension between matter and spirit. However, recall... that matter and spirit are not just opposites, but a duality. They are, therefore, complementary opposites. The tension between matter and spirit is a creative one, one that has the capacity to nourish us. But because so many people feel primarily fragmented by this tension, it's natural to wonder whether humanity is not meant to be much further along in the process of integrating matter and spirit than it is. Can we point to specific historical events that somehow resulted in humanity's being spiritually detoured?

Indeed, there are two historical factors which together have significantly delayed humanity's progress in unifying matter and spirit. The first of these factors is Jesus' physical death before he was able to set up a systematic method for transmitting certain information and energy initiations from one generation to the next—gifts that he wished to bequeath to humanity. To appreciate the last statement, we need to understand the difference between the mainstream or exoteric Christian interpretation of Jesus and the esoteric interpretation of Jesus. In the mainstream Christian interpretation Jesus is uniquely the Son of God who came to be [the] people's savior. In the esoteric interpretation, all of us are equally sons or daughters of God, and Jesus' mission, through his teachings and an esoteric system of initiation, was to facilitate people's ability to access the higher states of consciousness known in the west as Christ Consciousness....

In one esoteric interpretation, Jesus' physical death was not part of a divine plan for human salvation because it could not have been foreseen with absolute certainty. Human beings have free will, and this included the particular individuals responsible for Jesus' physical death. Certainly, if Jesus came to teach us that we are all equally children of God, then the mainstream Christian interpretation of God sacrificing an only son needs to change. In actuality, Jesus' physical death was premature and prevented him from establishing the Shakti lineage that he intended. It is true, as some have claimed, that part of Jesus' original esoteric teachings and initiations have survived; but they exist only in fragmented form, not as a whole and coherent system.

The energies that Jesus meant to bequeath were inspired variations of energies from the Jewish mystical tradition of Kabbalah, to which he was heir. In addition to being a spiritual genius, Jesus was also a Kabbalistic genius with deep and original insights into the energies used in his time. He saw, even though Kabbalistic energies were thought to be governed primarily by the metaphysical fire element, that the metaphysical water element had a much greater part in the operation of these energies than previously supposed. For example, the water component is responsible for the characteristic way that many Kabbalistic energies gradually integrate deeper and deeper into the Earth. Following divine guidance, Jesus cooperated with a consortium of many non-terrestrial masters, including those from Rigel, Betelgeuse, and Sirius, to create a system of Kabbalistic initiation that emphasized fire and water equally.

In his public ministry Jesus tried to develop in people the quality that has been called "Divine Vision," the ability to see the world more in the way that God sees it. For example, those with Divine Vision see all people as equally the children of God and see the loving support of God throughout nature. The main way that Jesus taught was through parables, which are attempts to wake us up from the trance induced by worldly concerns and to see and feel the reality of God's unconditional love for us. Jesus' concern with developing Divine Vision also greatly influenced the Kabbalistic system of initiation that he helped to co-create. A key part of that initiatory system was a Kabbalistic shakti that developed both Divine Vision as well as the capacity to feel God's loving presence in one's body. Jesus called this energy "The Foundation," both because it was one of the foundations of the system and also because he believed Divine Vision should be the foundation from which all of our actions stem. This energy is one of the main gifts that he intended to bequeath to humanity; however, he died prematurely before he could set up a lineage for the transmission of either this energy or the rest of his system.

Following Jesus' physical death, the Earth's Spiritual Hierarchy and the cooperating non-terrestrial masters could not find anyone with the genius to understand his system or with the charisma to set up a lineage with worldwide influence. If masters want to send energy to help humanity they can do it in two ways: either through energies that are meant to be communicated to people directly in initiations or through energies that are sent to the Earth's gridwork and which thus reach people indirectly. Although the gridwork approach affects human spiritual evolution much more slowly, this was the only approach available to the masters for getting Jesus' energies to humanity following his physical death. These energies are vital if humanity is to fully develop Divine Vision, the integration of matter and spirit, and those states known in the West as Christ Consciousness.

We want to emphasize that there are many beautiful and spiritually transformative energies from many traditions that have been present throughout history and continue to be present today. **We are not saying that Jesus' energies are the only ones, nor are we saying that they are the most important ones.** Their primary significance at this point in time comes from the fact that they are missing; that they are not present in the earth's gridwork system or in our subtle bodies to the degree they would be if Jesus' system had been passed on.

The fact that Jesus' energies were not passed on as a system of initiation is the first of the two historical factors reffered to above. The second factor has to do with the history of a secret guild of spiritually developed humans called "Earth Keepers." Throughout history these Earth Keepers have existed in cultures all over the world and have had the responsibility of helping to maintain the welfare of the Earth's subtle energy gridwork system, as well as adding new energies to facilitate the spiritual evolution of humanity. The Earth Keepers, put into the Earth's gridwork both energies received from previous generations of their guild as well as energies received from terrestrial and non-terrestrial masters.

One of the main reasons they have worked in secret is that the energies they use, like many advanced spiritual energies, can develop supernormal powers. The number of Earth Keepers at any given time has always been relatively small because each generation has difficulty in finding successors who are both talented enough and can also be trusted with the supernormal powers. However, even though their number is small, the presence of these Earth Keepers is critical because certain frequencies of energy can be placed into the gridwork only by physically-embodied beings.

Many advanced spiritual energies cannot be safely present in the Earth's gridwork system unless that system is sufficiently strong. One of the factors affecting the Spiritual Hierarchy's ability to continue sending Jesus' frequencies to the Earth's gridwork after his transition was the combined effort of the Earth Keepers in many lands. These Earth Keepers, with the help of the Office of the Christ, continuously strengthened the Earth's gridwork to hold higher and higher levels of Jesus' energies. Since Jesus' system consists of a graduated sequence of higher and higher frequencies, the vibration of the Earth's gridwork must be stepped up before each subsequent frequency level can be integrated.

A Key event in the history of the Earth Keepers occurred after the Romans invaded Celtic Britain in 43 A.D. By the time the Romans eventually left in 410 A.D., they had effectively destroyed Celtic civilization as it had previously existed. Very sadly, only a few generations after the initial Roman invasion, the Celtic branch of the Earth Keepers no longer existed. Many were killed by Romans, and the few who remained very reluctantly chose not to leave successors rather than pass their knowledge to those who could not be trusted with the development of supernormal powers.

Following the physical death of Jesus, even though his system was no longer available in human initiations, many terrestrial and non-terrestrial masters began the process of putting these key frequencies into the Earth's gridwork. Then gradually, over time, they began building up the levels of these needed frequencies. Following the demise of the Celtic Earth Keepers, the levels of Jesus' energies that were already in the gridwork system remained present, but gridwork lacked additional ongoing frequency upgrades necessary for higher vibration levels. Consequently, the cumulative effect of Jesus' premature transition and the demise of the Celtic Earth Keepers have significantly slowed the evolution of humanity's ability to integrate matter and spirit. Again, we are not saying that Jesus' energies are the only ones that can develop this ability; nor are we saying that they are the most important. The emphasis is on the fact that the higher levels of these energies are missing. *A key concept here is that the combined presence of energies from many different spiritual traditions, both in the Earth's gridwork and in our subtle bodies, is required before humanity can reach the highest stages of spiritual evolution.*

The story does not end here! The message... is really one of hope because events will soon take a much more positive turn. For many centuries the masters have had an ongoing project of finding ways to substitute for the missing frequencies of the Celtic Earth Keepers and of developing alternative paths for strengthening the gridwork's capacity to receive new and higher levels of Jesus' missing frequencies. *The good news is that this project will be completed in the year 2012 A.D.!* At that time there will also be one or more spiritual groups present who will be capable of restoring initiations with Jesus' original Foundation energy. The changes in the Earth's gridwork and the restoration of this particular part of Jesus' system will greatly accelerate humanity's spiritual evolution, including the critical capacity to integrate matter and spirit. It will also prepare the way for the appearance of the spiritual leader who has been called the World Teacher and the even greater transformation that he or she will bring.

As mentioned, many of the world's traditions are awaiting the predicted appearance of a major spiritual leader. Buddhists are waiting for Maitreya Buddha, Muslims are awaiting the Imam Mahdi, Jews are awaiting the Messiah, and Christians are awaiting the Christ. The truth is that all of these leaders are the same figure. This World Teacher will appear not just for the people of one particular faith, but will come for people of all faiths, as well as for those who have no spiritual beliefs.

This great being will be a new spiritual teacher rather than a former spiritual teacher reappearing.

*The World Teacher will coordinate the efforts of many people and masters to bring about a Golden Era of peace, justice, and harmony for humanity. Through an extraordinarily profound connection to the Earth's gridwork system, the World Teacher will act as a conduit for a great influx of energies to the Earth and humanity from many terrestrial and non-terrestrial masters. **The World Teacher will also institute a system of energy initiations that will unify the energies from all of the world's spiritual traditions.** He or she will also introduce those energies needed to inaugurate the next cycle of the Divine plan.*

It's important to understand that the World Teacher will be a spiritual leader, not political one, and will possess authority only to the extent that people voluntarily give it. It is also important to understand that the World Teacher will not be some sort of spiritual king, but more like the head of a committee. To use another analogy, the World Teacher will have a relationship to humanity and the Earth that is similar to the relationship of a person's crown chakra to their entire chakra system. The Golden Era of humanity cannot be brought about by one person no matter how powerful, but requires the coordinated efforts of all of us working together. (209-215)

VE[3]: *I'm sure that many ... will feel that your explanation about Jesus' transition ... detracts from the stature of Jesus. How could such a premature transition even happen to someone of Jesus' extraordinary power, love and wisdom? How could such a transition be consistent with the will of God?*

IF: *As someone who has the utmost respect for Jesus, I've certainly had to consider for myself the questions you just raised. I believe the information ... is completely consistent with having a special reverence for Jesus.*

Let me answer your first question about how a premature transition could have happened to someone of Jesus' extraordinary power, love, and wisdom. It is critical to understand that, as long as Jesus was present here on the earth in a physical body, his life was impacted by the free will decisions of others. God has given the inviolable attribute of free will to all human beings, including the particular individuals responsible for the arrest and crucifixion of Jesus.

Why were these individuals so opposed to Jesus in the first place? Great spiritual leaders have a way of antagonizing those who wish to place world concerns over the spiritual. For example, the Buddha and Mohammed each had more than one assassination attempt made on their lives. Quite aside from the fact that such leaders can threaten existing political power, D.K.[4] *tells us that the energy field of any master can be very disturbing to those who are not prepared to grow spiritually. The energy field of Jesus was especially powerful. For one thing he was continuously emitting energies of Divine Vision and these energies can be particularly disturbing, because as they open your vision they can cause you to question all of your values and all that you have done in a whole lifetime. ...*

The antagonism which Jesus aroused was so great and eventually became so organized that the only way he could have overcome it was by being responsible, either directly or indirectly, for the deaths of others. His moral code prevented him from doing this. Therefore, his physical death should not be seen as a defeat, but rather as a victory because he was willing for his physical body to perish rather than violate his deeply-held beliefs about nonviolence.

Appendix F

I believe Jesus' willingness to have his physical body perish was consistent with God's will. I do not believe that it was God's intention that Jesus die on the cross from the beginning. I believe it was God's original intention that people follow Jesus, not kill him. However, I believe the decision Jesus made to go on the cross, after he was arrested and imprisoned by the Romans, did represent God's will. It is useful to distinguish, as a number of theologians have, between God's antecedent will and God's consequent will. **Antecedent** *will refers to God's original intention with respect to a given situation, whereas* **consequent** *will refers to God's intention after the situation has been altered by the free will actions of human beings.*

I emphasize again that Jesus' death should not be seen as a defeat. We should see the opposition he aroused as a testament to his power and see his willingness to go to his death rather than desert his belief in nonviolence as a testament to the purity of his actions and belief. (216-217)

VE: *What is the position of Christianity today in terms of aiding the appearance of the next World Teacher?*

IF: *Those of the many Christian denominations that pass on true spiritual teachings are helping to prepare for the appearance of the World Teacher, as are all genuine spiritual teachings of all faiths. However, modern mainstream Christianity is doing nothing at all from an* **energetic perspective** *to prepare for the coming of the World Teacher. As mentioned, one of the great tragedies in the history of Christianity is the loss of the systematic passing on of the esoteric teachings and energies of Jesus. Fortunately, these teachings and energies have not been completely lost. Fragments do survive in scattered locations of the globe even though they have been lost as a coherent system.*

One of the important things to understand about any great spiritual leader is that such a leader always passes on both exoteric, or outer teachings, and esoteric, or inner teachings. Any teacher of any subject who is a good teacher will teach different people in different ways depending on their level of consciousness and willingness.

It's also important to understand that the purpose of the esoteric teachings is not to create some kind of an elite. Esoteric teachings are a natural outgrowth of this universal principle of good teaching as well as several other important facts. One is that some of the most important truths about the universe are difficult to believe when you first hear them, and if they are revealed prematurely, a person is likely to reject a truth that is very important for their development. The second point to understand about esoteric spiritual teachings, which distinguishes them from purely intellectual pursuits, is that advanced spiritual practices can lead to the development of various supernormal powers which a good spiritual teacher does not want to pass on indiscriminately.

Esoteric teachings exist in all great spiritual traditions, and even in the New Testament we see places where Jesus tells things to the disciples that he does not tell to the general public. So part of the tragedy of current Christianity is that in an admirable attempt to be democratic—this attempt coming from the recognition that all of us are equal before God—people have corrupted and disempowered the original Christian teachings by denying their esoteric component. But this need not be a permanent situation because the spiritual forces that are guiding humanity are hoping that the full esoteric teachings that Jesus meant to pass on can be brought back.... (218-219)

VE: *Can you say more about why our beautiful planet's gridwork is incomplete and has been weakened—to our disadvantage?*

IF: *The gridwork as it now exists is seriously incomplete because necessary frequencies are missing due to a series of interrelated historical calamities. One of these involves the demise of the Celtic Earth Keepers, as previously mentioned. The Celtic Earth Keepers also used chanting and toning to bring in divine, subtle sound frequencies. They knew how to utilize Stonehenge to spread those frequencies throughout the planet's gridwork system. There were also other frequencies missing due to misuses of powers in ancient Egypt, which caused the subsequent withdrawal of certain initiations by the Spiritual Hierarchy. A series of calamities also occurred that preceded Egypt, going back to ancient Lemuria and Atlantis. That's really where the problems with earth's gridwork started. Subsequent events, from ancient Egypt to modern times, are like knocking over of a row of karmic dominoes set up in ancient Lemuria and Atlantis.*

VE: *So these damages to the gridwork affected human consciousness and their ability to use energies appropriately.*

IF: *Absolutely, and the missing frequencies in the Earth's gridwork system affect us all in our daily lives very profoundly, in ways that most people don't realize. Many people who are sensitive to energy have the feeling that there's something missing, that their energy body is not quite right, and that this lack goes deeper than the influences of their family of origin and of the society in which they now live. It's very important to understand that although our subtle bodies are made up of subtle matter, it is still matter and it must be renewed and replenished! In our physical body we know that cells divide and that we produce new cells as a result of the food that we eat. In a similar way, the subtle bodies have matter that is subject to the law of entropy and over time degrades and must be replaced. Where does this replenishment come from?*

Let's take a look at the subtle mental body as an example. Most of the matter in our mental body is made from energy that we absorb from the Sun. The second most significant source of the matter in our mental body comes from trees, and there's a very profound connection between human mental bodies and the subtle energy field of trees. Many people sense this at an intuitive level. They know that when they are next to a tree their thinking is clearer and they feel more at peace. Because there are frequencies missing from the Earth's gridwork system, there are also very important frequencies missing from the energy fields of trees. Consequently, there are necessary frequencies missing from our mental bodies. Though most people aren't sensitive enough to energy to realize that something is missing, many people are, and that number is increasing...

IF: *...And it is...[also] true that trees...have a profound effect on our emotional bodies. Indeed, there are these very intimate links that exist between the different kingdoms of nature—between the mineral kingdom, the animal kingdom, the plant kingdom, and the human kingdom—which must not be disrupted. People are becoming familiar with the concept of ecology on a physical level, and in a similar way realize you can't disrupt the subtle energy fields of any one kingdom without affecting all kingdoms.*

VE: *So our feelings that we're not as powerful as we should be, that we can't do all the things that we'd like to do, not only come from what you would call a psychological lack of worth and so on, but from a very deep inner sensory level dissatisfaction. I hear many people saying how hard it is to be here on the planet knowing that they have something missing that can't quite be identified.*

IF: *Yes, many people have those feelings, and when they realize that there is some reason for them that can't be ascribed* to just their family of origin, their society of their environment—they often look for other reasons. These explanations might have to do with alien sources interfering with the Earth or something related to the DNA level. But the most important thing to emphasize is that the source of these feelings is not something exotic but is literally right under our feet. It's the very Earth—it's the water we drink and the air that we breathe—which lack certain energy frequencies. Indeed the reason these feelings can be so strong is beacuse this lack surounds us all the time in our daily life. We can't get away from the fact that everything we do is connected to Mother Earth.

These missing frequencies also influence people's spiritual development. Many people have had the experience of clearing themselves of certain negative thought forms only to have those return very quickly, leaving them at a loss to explain why is it so hard to remain clear of these unwanted thought forms. Of course, there are many reasons for this. However, one explanation is that our mental bodies are simply not as strong as they really should be at this point in time. If these missing frequencies were present in the Earth's gridwork and therefore in the trees and in our mental bodies, it would be much easier for people to clear negative thought forms out of their mental bodies. Then more often we would all feel the way that we do mentally and emotionally when we're in a forest, in nature....

IF: Indeed, as the Earth's missing frequencies are filled-in everyone will find it more joyful to be in a body. This will be particularly true for people who are consciously aware and sensitive to energy. There can be a real tendency for people to desire escaping from the body if they are sensitive to energy and notice the feeling that something is missing. However, the body is here for a reason, and we see that even when people evolve spiritually and become enlightened, they don't disappear in a puff of smoke or a flash of white light. They're still here in a body. *The **real purpose of humanity's spiritual evolution is not transcendence but wholeness. We are not here to abandon the body but to unify body and spirit.***

As the missing frequencies get restored to the Earth's gridwork it will become easier for people to enjoy the experience of being in a body. Let us be grateful that many masters are working to help bring about this shift in the Earth's gridwork and have been working at this for centuries. These include the masters of our own Planetary Hierarchy and many non-terrestrial masters.... When the World Teacher does appear the whole process of restoring Earth's missing frequencies will be greatly accelerated, for this is one of the functions of the World Teacher. It cannot be over emphasized that the World Teacher will come to develop a spirituality that links people even more deeply to the Earth and that increases people's appreciation for Mother Earth and their own bodies. (219-222)

VE: So what is the relationship between the World Teacher and the level of vibration of the Earth's grid and the people on the planet being able to receive this being's energy?

IF: The Earth's gridwork system has to be developed in two ways in order for the appearance of the World Teacher to occur. The first is that it must be strong enough to hold both the very high vibrational energies which will be emitted by the energy field of the World Teacher and the very high vibrational energies which the World Teacher will communicate through initiation to other people who will then carry them. The second point is that the gridwork must not only be strong enough to carry these energies, but it must also be able to ground the energies into the Physical Earth. Why? Because while these powerful energies will help humanity evolve, they're also coming to help ***nature*** evolve. These energies will actually shift the energy fields of many different plants and rocks, and those shifted fields will in turn affect the evolution of humanity. There are many intricate feedback loops here. So in order for the energy field of the Earth to be developed enough to ground the energies that will be emitted by the World Teacher, many subtle energy triangles have to be strengthened. As mentioned above, a particularly vital triangle is the one formed by the heart chakra of the Earth, the heart chakra of the Sun, and the heart chakra of Sirius. One of the critical functions of this essential triangle is to ground these energies that will be emitted by the World Teacher.

VE: Since we've talked so much about the changes that the World Teacher will bring, I need to suggest the possibility that the World Teacher could be a pair of beings or even a group of energies, not a single identity. And I should add that some people will undoubtedly disagree with the explanations concerning humanity's delayed spiritual progress. In any case I want to emphasize your previous point that the Golden Era of humanity cannot be brought in by efforts of just one person, no matter how powerful. Rather, this new era must come from the efforts of all of us cooperating together with the sometimes inscrutable cosmic rhythms and cycles which affect our lives so profoundly and continuously guide our destiny.... [And, indeed] the effectiveness of that cooperation is dependent on each of us continuing to work on our own personal and spiritual evolution....

It's vital to understand that spirit is always mediated through a particular form, and for us that form is presently a human body. Let us answer the age old calling to serve our Creator by using the physical form at our disposal with wisdom, compassion, and love. These characteristics are our cosmic passport beyond time and space, yet they must be gained by our willingness to seek them with our inner consciousness where they await unveiling and expression.

IF: Yes. And with all of this talk about what the future will bring, let us not forget the many blessings with which we have been endowed and which we can enjoy in current time. Surely one of these blessings is the stars. Like the person on the cover of this book, let us go into the night and raise our arms to the skies in celebration of their beauty and mystery. May we ever increase in knowledge and appreciation of their light and the light of the loving God who created them. (223-225)

Appendix G: Excerpts from *You Are Becoming a Galactic Human*[1]

I would want to ask you to reread my comments preceding the excerpts from Essene's Energy Blessings from the Stars in *Appendix F*. I have such a profound wish not to offer information that risks rejection because of my misjudgment in the timing of its presentation. All the same, it feels critical that we stretch our remembrancing at this time across the esoteric and the exoteric calendar of our evolution. So please then strive not to reject categorically those thoughts and possible truths that follow. Take rather those that resonate with you for yours and for your journey with them and place the others on a shelf in the storage spaces of your mind for further and/or later consideration as the future unfolds (Clark 125).

The text of the following *Appendix* is an assemblage of information selected from Virginia Essene's and Sheldon Nidle's presentation of the Galactic Federation's message for our planet — a volume that they have engagingly titled, You Are Becoming a Galactic Human. It is a collection of chaptered information from members of an emissary council of Sirians followed by questions posed by the two authors and answered by members of the council and most usually by a being named Washta — a galactic presence in the final phases of his training as a Sirian ascended master and indeed for whom training concludes with the completion of this verbal documentary of galactic purpose and intentionality. Virginia Essene's introductory chapter strikes me as a brilliant index both of the information to come and of the likely inner objections many may feel to this information. She encourages us each to evaluate for ourselves the information offered and she gives us five tools to help us in our efforts to remember

---

[1] Please see *Sources Cited* under Essene.

and to reconnect with our planet's history and with humanity's true origins. She asks in her book, New Cells, New Bodies, New Life!:

> Is it possible that in some encoded but suspended animation, we have held the memory of our original genetic origin and its awesome capabilities until we could evolve back in our consciousness?[2] Is this the present momentous experience in which our inner waters — beyond blood to the flowing electromagnetic energy of molecular life — can be reclaimed? (Essene, You Are Becoming 3)

And to these questions her overwhelming "YES" wells up — exquisitely resonant and wonderfully known from within. She supplements her "YES" with a flowing index of earlier phases of Earth's history (Lemurian and Atlantean civilizations for example) on through chronicles of our DNA's mutation, the Biblical flood, contemporary Catholicism and other Christian and eastern cosmologies. In passing, Essene points out the similarities of tales from Sumerian, Egyptian, Zoroastrian, Semitic and Hindu texts and pictographic testimonials of extraterrestrial visitation replete with vehicles for interspatial travel and wars engaged in for the purpose of altering Earth's beings both genetically and behaviorally. Mayan, Incan, and Aztec mythologies are touched on as well as they echo the same themes.[3] Even in themselves the details of the historical continuum she creates and the similarities she notices would more than serve as a compelling invitation to scan her introduction in its entirety. The global cohesiveness it manages to portray might leave many of us attuned to the real harmonies of a vicarious knowingness of our communion, our unity, and our oneness — for sure a knowingness profoundly beyond any previously imagined or meditationed embrace of microcosm and macrocosm and of microcosm as macrocosm. She has not contented herself with the enormity of just this Sirian version of Earth's galactic history — choosing to include as well their glorious presentation of potential futures and Earth's role in such present and future tenses. These present and future tenses are deliciously cognizant of humanity's free will and present themselves as a collection of variable scenarios. All the same, they leave the reader comforted with a sense of galactic trust and knowingness that at least a portion of this planet and her people will make the constructive choices and energetic shifts that propel them towards that

---

[2] It is said that the Elohim, "mighty angels who embody high intelligence and creative powers, and who sit at the right hand of God himself" (Polich 31) were responsible for sending the many world teachers we've had over our planet's millennia — world teachers sent to help humanity awaken into higher states of spiritual consciousness (Polich 38). Among these teachers has been the great Egyptian named Thoth — and later known as Hermes Trismegistus by the Greeks — also Moses among the Hebrews, Quetzalcoatl in Central America, Vishu, Krishna, and Buddha in the East and Jesus of Christian lineage and Mohammed of Islamic heritage.

[3] ". . . Legends of a return to paradise or a golden age are found worldwide. They are an aspect of most religions and include the concept of Shambala, the return of the great white brother, the golden age that is to follow the Kali Yuga foretold in Hindu teaching; the golden age prophesied by the Andean Masters; and the regeneration of earthly paradise promised in Judeo-Christian teachings. It seems apparent that this is the time foretold in many legends and myths from around the world and in the sacred traditions of many indigenous peoples — the time of the great awakening." (Polich 102-103)

Appendix G

blessed embrace of their ultimate potential and their guardianship role in the evolution of their galaxy and their universe. Above all else I see the breadth of this information as abundantly fear-relieveing and disaster-consciousness reformatting — an esoteric and exoteric gift to us of that truth about ourselves that can allow us to know, to be, and to manifest our divinity and our potential:[4]

> ... *[Perhaps] Jesus' message was delivered to a society of human beings whose genes may have been damaged by the Atlantean genetic experiments thousands of years before his arrival.*
>
> *These people who lived in the Middle East were certainly courageous, and we probably cannot imagine the terrors they went through. But we see from present-day history that they were ignorant of their own local history—hardly cognizant of the Egyptian, Sumerian and Babylonian civilizations and their relationships with what we call star people or extraterrestrial visitors.*
>
> *That Middle East remnant was not only separated from their own full consciousness as human beings, but most of their regional history had been destroyed in the biblical flood so they had no records of what had gone before. Imagine what it would be life if, today, we had all of our personal and societal belongings and records destroyed. How long could we remember our past? Would it soon be forgotten except through oral stories and myths? How could human continuity be retained with distorted genetic codes?*
>
> *Because of that great watery inundation, then, those located in the Middle East lost whatever data they had known about themselves and also about the nations in Asia, especially the greatest of all Earth civilizations—Lemuria. Since they had lost virtually all knowledge of Lemuria, they also had lost the records of Lemuria's later adversary—Atlantis....*
>
> *... [H]uman knowledge about who we are was no longer remembered or even historically recorded. Nearly every morsel of information was lost to everyday mental recollection. Without their former psychic abilities, such as mental telepathy, seeing and hearing spiritual energies, communing with nature, and so forth, how could they now retrieve this former human history? Since ... [many of us] today are ... [not yet fully developed in our] psychic sensitivities of higher consciousness, the truth of who we are and why we are here is also still deeply hidden. That is why I believe we keep sensing there is a core of mystery that needs to be solved—the greatest human mystery of all times! A mystery daring us to remember and reclaim our original God-given nature....*
>
> *Although some individuals find a peace and joy to base their lives upon, others are racked with painful circumstances such as war, violence, and starvation. ... "Is it possible that in some encoded but suspended animation, we have held the memory of our original genetic origin and its awesome capabilities until we could evolve back in consciousness? Is this the present momentous experience in which our inner waters—beyond blood to the flowing electromagnetic energy of molecular life—can be reclaimed?"[5]*

---

[4] Free will and all (giggle giggle).

[5] Essene quoting in <u>You Are Becoming a Galactic Human Being</u> (3) from her book <u>New Cells, New Bodies New Life!</u>.

... "YES"... this is the time of that momentous experience when full molecular capability will be reclaimed! This is the historical juncture when we offspring of an awesome Creator reclaim the cellular credentials of galactic birthright. But to welcome the occasion with the vitality and assurance that it deserves, we must truly be willing to surrender our rigid earth-based history and look into the galactic history with which we are associated. (2-4)

Because many humans deny the indigenous people's valuable information and refuse to believe who the whales and dolphins really are, much of what we need to know is lost. Just as refusing to acknowledge our planet as a living being is a major error! But these three sources of assistance will be increasingly valuable in the days ahead if we will but open our minds to include them. Knowledge, safety and joy can be added to our lives as we awaken and consciously attune to all of them....

But can we hold onto love after we learn our true and hidden Earth history?... after we discover that we are mutant starseed creations?... and that there really has been a war in the lower realms where we exist? Can love then remain in our hearts? For love is the key to conscious reclamation of our higher origins and capabilities, and those who do not express love's powerful nature will not easily flow into the accelerated advancement humanity is now being offered by spirit and the galactic human family....

(Please feel comfortable in ignoring this challenge if you are not at ease with this exploration of new ideas and/or new perceptions of the old. Perhaps these new ideas or interpretations may not serve you just now. But if you feel the longing to explore human history more fully, come join our explorer's alliance....)

It is imperative that we do not feel guilty that our text books are inadequate, often mistaken, and generally incomplete at best. [And] just because there is little or no physical proof or evidence in the major sciences like biology, geology, anthropology, astronomy, and so on, it does not mean there has been no history (Essene, You Are Becoming 16). As researchers we are looking to find the gaps and fill them so others who don't have time to become thoughtful explorers can benefit from our contributions. Our love and willingness to learn will not only help ourselves, but others, as well. Therefore, this material is not just for us, personally, but for the planet and all of her other life forms! (5-6)

photon belt - questions and answers

Washta: ... Our present interest is but a continuation of the overseeing of your spiritual development—along with the cooperation of the spiritual hierarchies of your planet and the solar system—so present day Earth humans can acquire full consciousness once again. Secondly, we come to introduce the Galactic Federation that was created to bring the profound light of the Supreme Creative Force into this glorious galaxy.

We are therefore here in love and in light, to oversee, to aid, and one might say to midwife a new civilization. Those of us on this council are able and eager to do this task for we have been appointed by a higher council that might be called in your language, ascended masters, and in our language (as translated into English), galactic presences.

We, and beings from many higher levels of existence, have interacted with other various ascended masters, angels and archangels of many dimensional realms of this physical universe on your behalf. They are all helping to create a new energy of love and wisdom across this entire galaxy because the time has now come again for your planet to belong to this diverse galactic family. Yes, you are to experience this great leap forward into a new Age of Light and to let the interdimensional Christ Consciousness touch you more fully. This Christ Consciousness originates from the very core of creation to this world. It comes so that more love and light can now be brought to full consciousness, and so that all men and women on your planet can act as guardians for planet Earth and its accompanying solar system.

... [T]he photon belt itself could be called "the great light that is coming." Photon is a particular kind of energy you haven't identified as yet. Right now, the photon belt energies are located at an angle where they are very difficult to be seen except by very powerful astronomical instruments. The governments of your planet have largely prevented those who have access to such instruments from sharing their findings in the public light. This suppression has led to a great deal of confusion among those who have been given information about its true cause and nature. Since your instruments are still very limited in properly identifying photon energy, just think of it as the great light that has been talked about in many prophecies, by many peoples throughout the past few thousand years of recorded human history on your planet....

... It is a lower vibratory level of the energies of pure God light; however, it is still a great celestial energy. It was put into place for the purpose of bringing various star systems into alterations of consciousness, of bringing them through changes and shifts in dimensions. This is what is going to occur here once again on Earth. You are about to re-experience this drama that the Earth and its solar system have entered many times, because there is roughly a 26,000 year cycle involved in this whole process.

The last photon belt experience happened around the time of the destruction of Lemuria, approximately 25,000 years ago; however, it was not the cause of that destruction as we will later explain.

It is an energy that operates in a 3rd- and a 4th-dimensional reality. It is a great energy of light that changes and alters itself and creates great openings into dimensional time portals—which is what the 4th dimension is about. Therefore, whenever the Earth and your solar system go through the photon belt's alterations, great shifts occur in the radioactive activities of your planet and in its electrical and magnetic fields. Some shifts have occurred that have caused great catastrophes so it is basically what one might call an awesome omen of change in the sky which your planet has passed through from time to time. (44-46)

Virginia: ... Please further clarify why Earth's human family and the planet are being helped at this particular time.

Washta: The first reason is the great increase humans made in consciousness, beginning in the 1950s, accelerating in the 1960s and the 1970s— and most especially in the late 1980s. Secondly, because the Spiritual Hierarchy of Lady Gaia (the name we give to the Earth and all of its angels, archangels and ascended masters) decided to save your planet's civilization, contrary to the Galactic Federation's Sirian Regional Council's opinion. The cetaceans and the Earth's Spiritual Hierarchy first requested, back in the early 1970s, that some of the solar difficulties of this particular cycle of the photon belt experience be alleviated for your civilization.

We, Sirians, are deeply committed to aid the Spiritual Hierarchy of your planet and solar system and always do what we feel is desired by the great will of the God Force. Therefore, we began petitioning on your behalf among other council members within the Galactic Federation's Sirian Regional Council to protect your physical world from the unspeakable catastrophe that would surely occur because of the upcoming photon belt. The photon belt would have created the great catastrophic scenario that many of your psychics have been warning about during the last decade and a half. However, because of the intervention of the Earth's Spiritual Hierarchy and because of the rise in human consciousness since the 1950s, this new scenario was given priority and is now being implemented....

... You see, many members in the Galactic Federation's Sirian Regional Council (that have jurisdiction over your particular planet and solar system) had previously agreed that it was necessary for humans to experience the photon belt. This was because the mutant human civilization on your planet was not raising its consciousness to the desired level—a level required for it to be saved on a mass basis. However, because of the intervention of the Spiritual Hierarchies (including your great spiritual leaders such as Lord Jesus, etc.), the intervention of the cetaceans, as well as we Sirians pleading on your behalf with the Galactic Federation—Sirian Regional Council members allowed this dreadful photon belt to be shifted after voting for the adoption of the present positive plan we bring. (47-48)

Washta: Let us clarify that the incoming photon belt is causing a great deal of stress on your entire solar system, not merely planet Earth. However, you have three levels of assistance helping you with this problem. One comes from the great spiritual caregivers and angels on many different dimensions. A second comes from those in human form who assist the God forces. And then, of course, we have been aiding you by instituting protective energy patterns around your planet. This enormous, combined effort keeps the amount of seismic activity to a minimum. This is why various earthquakes around your planet have not been as dangerous in magnitude as they could have been.

However, while seismic activity on your planet will be kept as low as possible, there must be some activity for there is a natural energy release pattern that Earth normally goes through. And humans have done destructive bombings above and below ground that have taken their toll, have they not? Some humans on this planet may experience death or dislocation in spite of our best efforts because there are some poorer countries where the housing structures and public buildings cannot withstand even the smallest tremors. This is because they are inexpensively constructed or improperly erected to resist earth movement. We regret that any loss of life as a natural act of nature must happen and assure you we are doing amazing things to minimize what would otherwise be a near total planetary disaster!

Virginia: Yes and we thank you for that help and concern! Nonetheless, can you imagine what the average human person thinks who hears you say that the Galactic Federation scientists are able to do something so powerful as to realign the Sun? To most of us, the Sun is such a major aspect of life that it seems permanent, or at least available for billions of years. Could you just briefly describe how such a seemingly unbelievable thing was accomplished?

Washta: The explanation is as follows: All celestial objects, or heavenly bodies, as they are called in your basic science, have interdimensional portals around them. These exist in various angles around the entire orb. For example, the Sun—which is the one you wish to discuss—is a very special star for Earth's existence, but it is a star nonetheless. As a star, it has a longevity much as every human on your planet has one. Because the Sun is now in what might be called a later middle-age period, it has already matured, so to speak, and has established these energy portals. These energy portals control its very existence—in fact, physical planets and stars like your Sun are a different life form than what you presently think. They are a new type of living organism that you will learn about as your science increases its willingness to know the truth.

You will begin to understand that what I am about to say is not only logical but simple science. How one goes about the entire process is as follows. First, the energy portal points on a particular star are energized and examined. Then once the degree of imbalance is completely analyzed, one can then set apart various counter energy points in these portals. When the Sun's energy portals are activated, these energy patterns then flash over it in a vast high frequency light across the entire solar magnetosphere—which extends out and includes its entire solar system, all its planets, its asteroids, its comets, etc. Basically, this is what was done. We could explain this in greater detail, but would like to keep our explanation simple and avoid advanced mathematics. . . .

. . . [M]aneuvers—concerning the positive alteration of your Sun—required not only our science but also the great intervention of the Spiritual Hierarchies. These Spiritual Hierarchies control the 3rd, 4th, and 5th interdimensional portals (gates) that surround your Sun. Once these maneuvers were completed, the final stages of these positive alterations could proceed.

Virginia: . . . Is there any way that our Earth scientists would be able to determine that this is now a different kind of Sun than what they could view astronomically in prior times?

Washta: They would notice that the star they called the Sun has gone through vast changes in its magnetosphere, that its cronosphere has greatly changed and that Sun spot activity patterns have been altered. These phenomena occurred because they are the physical manifestations of the interdimensional shifts that were required to bring the Sun and its great promenades under control, thus avoiding a near disaster for your planet. We interceded so that your planet and solar system could gradually move toward that photon belt and the safer destiny recommended by your Spiritual Hierarchy. Know that angels, spiritual masters, the Time Lords, and ultimately the great God Force itself, have saved your planet through this process. . . .

Washta: Those of the dark forces, as you call them, did not want the transformation of humanity to occur nor did they want us to bring this entire solar system into the light. They attempted to interfere with the Sun in such a way as to cause its entire system to be vastly altered—so that their reality could determine the future destiny of the entire solar system. Therefore, our intervention was required since it had been agreed by the Earth's Spiritual Hierarchies that whatever happened to your planet must be done within its own destiny patterns, not those patterns brought from some other place.

So we Sirians, along with the Galactic Federation, brought in those of science and a pure spirit to alter this entire system. The result is that your planet now sits in the midst of a hologram causing your reality to appear to be unchanged. However, a vast shift has already occurred because of Galactic Federation intervention, though you don't know it yet. What is now happening to you is unprecedented but protects you from psychological overload and distress. Within the planetary hologram you are being allowed to gradually move through changes and shifts in reality. These changes will allow you to reclaim what was meant to be your destiny as a fully conscious person in a civilization existing within a fully conscious, multidimensional world. (49-51)

Virginia: The average person who thinks about the Sun probably thinks about the words heat and light. Has there been any shift or change in what we would call the Sun's output of heat or light?

Washta: Heat and light from the Sun have been changed because portions of its energy have been drawn off to support this new hologram placed around your entire solar system. This hologram will protect you when your planet goes into the photon belt which is why we say the polarity energies of the Sun have been altered. This has been done in order to obtain the successful completion of the great shift in reality that is about to happen on your world. (52)

Virginia: We are concerned about the process of safely guiding people—especially children—through the photon belt experience.... [W]e feel that there hasn't been the kind of preparation from our governments that would allow people to believe in the process and begin to prepare for it. We wonder if you have any further comments, suggestions or recommendations about how this could best be dealt with?

Washta: We would ask that all people who are engaged in lightwork of any type whether it is with the angelic or guardian groups, whether with ecological difficulties, with the cetaceans, or any aspects of human development and preservation of life whatsoever, come together and network among themselves. By sharing the latest news among themselves and then sharing with others around them, all people on your planet who have access to the light networks can be prepared. In this way you can act as a prototype.

We would also ask of you who form these networks to come together and establish dates and times to do your meditations. Also formulate actions based upon your cooperative consciousness that will give you comfort and security. Be prepared to act in unison for the good of humanity in thought and deed! For it will not take a huge number of humans, acting as a unified group around your globe, to bring this great energy of change and consciousness to the planet and allow it to be safely anchored in such a way that it supports everyone—even those who still sit in denial of it.

Virginia: Thank you, and that brings to mind one last major question. Some people believe there has been a karmic requirement for people to become conscious through their own growth and education, and others believe that grace, as we understand it, allows total forgiveness and love to be granted to all—thereby canceling out all karma and negativity. Is it possible for this kind of grace to be applied to over 5 billion people on Earth? Have you any final thoughts or explanation concerning this issue of karma and grace?

Washta: We would like to state first of all, to all beings who reside on planet Earth in human form, that your planet is a planet of grace. It is a planet in which all who have incarnated on it, have done so because of this opportunity of grace and forgiveness. This law of love and light is the basis of the Spiritual Hierarchy and all that is created in and around it. Earth humans must realize that they came here to Earth to put this love and light, this grace of forgiveness, around this entire planet. They will realize as your world ascends, that humans came to Earth for this purpose. For as the consciousness falls on the planet and then rises into the great light around it, the amnesia which has prevented humans from seeing this light will be lifted. One might use the analogy of a blind man who suddenly falls down, hurting his head. But to everyone's amazement, he discovers that the accident has miraculously given his sight back. This miracle is what is about to happen to you and your *planet. You are about to come out of the darkness and blindness into light—into a stunning and incredible vision.*

Virginia: *In other words, the prior state of our consciousness does not count for, or against, having our consciousness raised through the photon belt experience?*

Washta: *That is absolutely correct. Earth is a planet of grace. It is becoming a planet that will truly demonstrate this grace and love, so everyone who is a part of this galaxy can come here to observe the results and to realize that your model can spread to every part of this great galaxy.*

Virginia: *So we would become as galactic humans going forth as a model for other planets and star systems?*

Washta: *That is correct. This star—your planet—was put in this universe and this galaxy for the purpose of becoming one of the great showcases or models of light. It is to be a major focal point or example of light, love and forgiveness for this entire galaxy. By your example many of the undecided or the dark beings will see the actual application of the Creator Force's grace so they, too, may ascend into the energy of the Time Lords. They too may enter that timeless realm of light that is truly a heavenly one, as described in many prophecies that now exist around your present human civilization. This is what your planet is about. This is the great mission of your world and of humans on the planet. You are about to enter into the age when your destiny will be fulfilled....*

... We would just like to finish with one final thought. We would ask all on your planet to realize that there is a new age of consciousness growing on planet Earth. At present, in fact, every human on planet Earth is being altered genetically, some in very small ways, others in larger ways, depending upon the position that they must play in bringing this great new civilization into reality. You of this world are seeking, as never before, to understand what the energy is that surrounds you. This is part of the pattern of bringing this new energy of consciousness back into human civilization and allowing it to alter your civilization as it has not been altered for vast millennia. Therefore, please cooperate with this new galactic civilization. What we are doing is no more than bringing this energy in with the assistance and full love of the cetaceans, and also the will of the Spiritual Hierarchy that is surrounding your planet. We ask you to realize that what is happening is not something to fear. Rather, it is a gift of love, light, and grace leading to a great and glorious destiny for Earth's awakening prodigals. (54-56)

the photon belt's effect on the human body

... [Let us next consider] what the photon belt's effect will be on the human body, particularly; and explain what this will mean to your planet and your civilization as well.... [T]he physical body of all Earth human beings will be completely altered as a result of the coming photon belt. Humans will be changed from having a gross or dense physical body to a semi-etheric or less dense one. At present, all body types are relegated by researchers in this field of somatic research into three major categories. These body types are as follows: 1) a gross or very physical body (your present 3rd-dimensional body type), 2) an etheric body (similar to auras, ghosts or to higher dimensional bodies), and 3) a purely spiritual body (the so-called soul body). Let us look at the consequences of this change for your body.

The first type—the physical body—is what most Earth humans of this planet are presently encased in. This body type consists of a flesh and blood physique that ages and eventually dies after a relatively short period of but five, six, seven, eight, or possibly nine or ten decades. What will happen in the coming galactic civilization is a transformation of this presently gross or physical body into a more etheric body that we will call a semi-etheric body. This body type is one that has the capabilities and appearance of the present physical body but with many of the characteristics possessed by a purely etheric body.

... Your semi-etheric body will respond in many ways like a thought form because your mind will be able to change your body as easily as it changes thoughts. However to you, this body will appear and act as if it were still the original type of gross physical body that you have now. Moreover, this new body will have still another dramatic transformation. This fundamental modification has to do with the composition of your DNA....

... [W]e are helping your DNA coils increase from two to twelve (or six fold) again. This transformation will restore the cellular structure of the body to its original form and allow the cells in your body to easily interact with the interdimensional spirit body (soul) that it contains.... This new configuration will follow the shape of a "Star of David" and allow each cell to easily connect to its topographical counterpoint on other dimensional levels.... The cell will thus possess a multidimensional scalar wave antenna that can easily pick up and immediately process any important message that the cell and its DNA package are given by the soul. Scalar waves are non-hertzian wave forms that have the ability to propagate themselves in any form of multidimensional reality and carry information with them as they travel. Similarly, your body will also change in the way its chakra centers (energy vortexes) are put together. (57-58)

your new chakra system / semi-etheric body

In your new semi-etheric body, a great deal of variation will occur on how these energy centers operate and how they will interact with one another (62).

... [Y]our chakras will be converted from the seven centers you now have to eleven human centers. [See Figure 9.] These additional four centers will interlink with two interdimensional or etheric centers at the top of your auric field that are called the galactic male and galactic female centers. In effect, you will have a total of thirteen chakras. Two of them will be purely etheric in form and eleven will become a part of your physical selves....

The **first chakra** will be in the same place as it previously was and will still be called the root center.

The **second chakra** will also remain as the sexual or sex center.

The **third chakra** will continue as the solar plexus center.

The **fourth chakra** is the first major modification. It will now be called the diaphragm center. This new chakra will be the center for governing stress since it will be the focal point for rejuvenating the prana or breath energy of the body. The prana or energy of the air acts to revitalize the body and to remove all deleterious elements from the body.

The **fifth chakra** becomes the heart center. It is not just a center for intuitive energy and higher emotions such as love; but it has also become a center for the expression of pure angelic love that is devoid of all base emotional expression.

Because your body has been changed from a purely physical form to a somewhat more etheric thought form, it will have an exceptional immune system that is extremely strong and viable. You will use the **sixth chakra** *or thymus center to act as the focus of all these activities. The thymus gland is presently one of the most misunderstood glands of the human body. This paradox concerns the thymus' sensitivity to radiation. The high levels of radiation in your planet's atmosphere that create aging were produced when it was ripped asunder by catastrophic events during your antediluvian histories about 6,000 years ago (see chapters 5 and 6). This radiation caused the thymus center in humans to rapidly deteriorate by early childhood and to shrink from an organ almost the size of the human heart to an organ about the size of a small pea.*

As the new human body advances to galactic form after the photon belt's arrival, the thymus will only shrink from the size of your present human heart to a size about one-third of the human heart. What this means is that your thymus center will remain as active and as virile in the adult body as it was in the body of a newborn. The ability of the human body to ward-off all kinds of diseases and any difficulties associated with the environment will, therefore, remain extremely high and the thymus will not shrink as one grows older. In other words, this new thymus center will make aging practically non-existent among galactic humans.

The **seventh chakra** *is the throat center and it is the center for communications and speech. This area will function in many of its former capacities because it is a conduit for the energies emanating from the head to the rest of the body.*

The **eighth chakra** *is called the well of dreams center. It is considered by many to be an old atrophied chakra and it is located roughly near the base of the skull, right above the neck. This chakra is needed to regulate the various dream and vision-like states that a fully conscious being can reach.*

The **ninth chakra** *develops into a control center for consciousness, and will be fully developed in the galactic human. It is located in the lower central part of the brain and consists of the so-called primitive brain and the pituitary gland. In a galactic human, it will allow the body to react to light and radiation in a way that permits the body to rejuvenate itself. The sixth chakra or thymus center and the ninth chakra or pituitary center interact with one another to heal and to revitalize the body.*

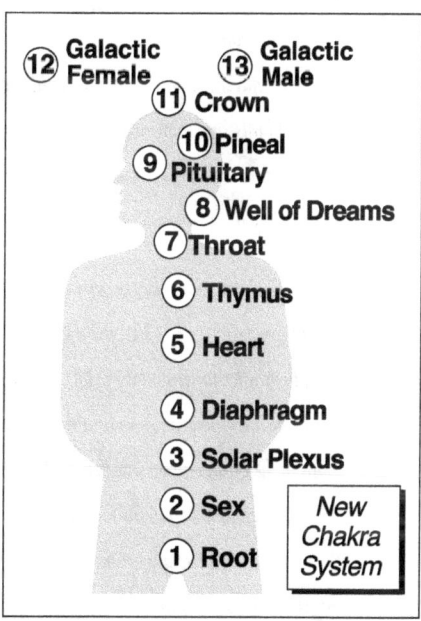

Figure 9: The New Chakra System[6]

The **tenth chakra** *will be known as the third eye or vision center, because it brings in the higher light frequencies. This chakra joins with the eighth chakra to allow the mind to interpret visions and other messages from higher vibratory states.*

The **eleventh chakra** *now assumes service as the crown chakra. It is where the physical body will connect to the spiritual energy, to invigorate your body. The crown is the place where the auric fields of the body come together making possible major*

---

[6] Essene, <u>You Are Becoming</u> 66.

connections to the **twelfth** and **thirteenth chakra** centers. These final two spiritual chakras are the *galactic male* and *galactic female energy centers* because they contain the ideal female and male prototype....

Because of these various changes to the chakra system, the many segments of the brain that were atrophied by Atlantean genetic experiments will be returned to their former shape and size. In two generations, humans will again have the larger style brain cavity that is the heritage of fully conscious humans. This will allow your scalar wave antenna to be fully utilized and all psychic energies to be processed in an appropriate manner. In effect, Earth humans will not only have first or primal sight, but also a complete "second sight" granting so many so-called psychic abilities such as telepathy, telekinesis, clairvoyance, and clairaudience....

... [Y]ou are moving from a 3rd dimensional physical reality to a 5th dimensional (semi-ethereal) reality. You are moving into a world in which all minds share a common consciousness and human beings no longer have the kind of separate world that you presently have. You are also moving to a consciousness where things can be done by humans that would, at present, be considered miraculous. Therefore, every Earth human must understand what his/her capabilities are and what his/her realities mean....

After you learn some basic qualities of galactic humanness, you can enjoy having a lighter body and using thought forms to rejuvenate and overcome aging. You will also have the ability to communicate within your own being, with other people, plants, and animals including Lady Gaia herself. You will also have full communication with those who have died in previous times as well as those who might today be called angels or archangels. In short, you will become both a being of spirit and a being of the physical. (65-70)

Washta: Most Earth scientists are only beginning to vaguely discover how the mind operates as a light or a holographic imprint unit. When the theta, or delta or the other dream-state wave patterns are in full focus, the mind is opening itself to its interdimensional portals. The scalar wave process, as it presently operates in the brain of Earth humans, requires complete unconsciousness so that the regular body functions can be lowered to minimal levels. In this way, the regular functions of the brain cannot interfere with scalar wave transmissions and reception. Using scalar wave functioning, the present brain's antenna is at a minimal efficiency.

In a fully conscious human, conversely, these scalar waves are already present in a fully conscious state. Therefore, lowering the body to a minimal level of function is not required. Hence, it is essential that one now realize a basic difference between Earth humans and fully conscious galactic humans. This difference is why most fully conscious humans do not require as much sleep as present Earth humans. The reason for this is that only when the body of an Earth human is in a minimal level (sleep) can it utilize this scalar wave. Once the scalar wave is utilized, the interdimensional brain functions can be used to bring-in data needed to control the processes of the mind and also of the different functions of the body.

These brain processing functions set up the next day's relationship between the various energy patterns in the body and the mind, and are done only when the Earth human is in a sleep state. In a fully conscious human, however, these functions can be accomplished in a fully awake state. Therefore, sleep to Earth humans is the regeneration mode. It is the way the body *assesses what is happening to it, what it needs to do in the next day, and how these developments relate to the physical body for an entire year, month, or a week of life. (71-72)*

Washta: *[Let us repeat, a] scalar wave is a non-hertzian frequency. It is propagated through interdimensional portholes and forms the basis of constituting all the various energies of creation. Scalar waves are what light comes from. It is that which makes all things in creation. It is based upon pulses that are called in the creation mythologies of the Galactic Federation, "the pulses of time"—for scalar waves are a timeless energy. This is what the human mind utilizes to provide the energies that make possible all aspects of physical existence....*

...Scalar waves are the scientific basis for all of those things that humans on your planet have given many different names. (75)

god and guardianship

...At present, and understandably so, Earth humans do not fully comprehend their new upcoming pattern....

Let's begin by looking at God's creation from a purely spiritual aspect. The Earth, as with all the various planets of the solar system, is surrounded by a Spiritual Hierarchy composed of spiritual beings called angels, archangels, and ascended masters. Their sole purpose is to act as spiritual mediators for the eight interdimensional evolutionary energies. These angelic mediators transfer these energies through the appropriate interdimensional portals for transport into your 3rd-dimensional stellar energy pattern. These creative and evolutionary energy patterns, in turn, create the physical universe which includes your solar system and the planet that you are now residing upon.

... This creation is one that is continuous and evolutionary in nature. Every aspect of a particular creation has an important and unique cycle. This present creation is the 6th cycle and will run between 50 billion to 100 billion years....

Some 50 billion years ago, your universe's physical creation was begun by the Time Lords under the direction of the Supreme Creative Force (God). This present creation is the last in a series of six creations that have continued from the beginning of time. Each physical creation had its own cycle and its own pattern. ***This physical creation was done to show how light could transmute darkness to produce an even higher light, which is composed of the highest love. This love will transform your galaxy and raise it towards the Supreme Creative Force and its chief emissaries, the Time Lords.*** *(139-140)*

Since you may not have heard of the Time Lords, we will describe them. They are what might be called the divine shepherds of ***physical creation***. *When the Supreme Creative Force first began the physical creation, the Time Lords were created, for time is the unit that controls all of physical creation.... The Time Lords exist in an infinite number of dimensions and their task is to regulate and to supervise the physical creation according to divine right action.*

Actually, the purpose of the Time Lords is two-fold in nature. Initially, they had to create the eight dimensions of physical creation, and secondly, they aided the dimensional Spiritual Hierarchies in their task of regulating the spiritual energy exchanges between each dimension. It is the task of the Spiritual Hierarchies to control interdimensional energy transfer by the use of interdimensional gates or, as they are also called, star gates. These gates serve as the flux barriers between dimensions and aid by regulating the energy flow to allow only those sufficient energy exchanges needed to successfully maintain the viability of physical creation. As a part of this divine plan, the Time Lords had to construct the 3rd-dimensional galaxy according to the divine plan of the Supreme Creative Force. To accomplish these tasks, the Time Lords were given the creative "pulse of time." With this energy tool, all things are possible and can be accomplished according to the divine plan. (140)

... [L]et us look at these eight dimensions from your point of view and get a better understanding of how reality is formulated. [See Figure 20.] The first seven dimensions are each created to express various aspects of the physical creation. The eighth level is the one where all of these lower qualities come from....

Let's discuss more about these seven dimensions. The first through the third dimensions are ones that you are well aware of. These dimensions are the physical realms that Earth science has long studied. Above them, there exists the 4th dimension which is a time portal through which the 3rd dimension passes into the 5th dimension. The 5th, 6th, and the 7th dimensions are what might be called higher dimensional realms and the laws of Earth science and physics do not therein apply.

To those who do not fully understand the science of the spirit, these levels might be comparatively viewed as lands of magic and miracles. Here in these higher realms, the spiritual beings called the angels and archangels of the Godhead exist. These angels and archangels, in turn, dwell in various levels of the Spiritual Hierarchy and are layered around the Earth in different dimension (5th, 6th, and 7th dimension) to protect it. The archangels and angels have a primary mission to perform—namely, to receive and to distribute the love and light energy of creation throughout the physical universe. The Time Lords, in turn, have a responsibility to monitor and continuously create the physical universe using the love and light energies given them in interdimensional exchanges by the Spiritual Hierarchy. The Spiritual Hierarchy members have a procedure that they follow to accomplish the interdimensional exchanges. They need in the physical realm, especially the 3rd dimension, a physical guardian who can perform their task of energy exchange on a smaller and more localized level, such as a star system or a planet. Therefore, **the physical guardians of any planet must be beings who are both physical and spiritual—in other words, physical beings who possess full consciousness.**

Let us look at planet Earth and begin to understand how this process is established. The devic aspect of the Spiritual Hierarchies has manifested the love and light energies that make the physical world possible. In effect, these devic spirits have manifested the physical energies that are necessary to sustain all life on Earth. They have established upon your planet a system of life which we call a specific biosphere. The purpose for life inhabiting a planet is two-fold. The first purpose of life is to manifest those specific energies that make any planet's existence even feasible. A second aim is to act in such a way that the various energies that are given life forms will be vivified and bring forth a continual growth in consciousness.

All animals, plants, rocks, water, sky, etc. have energies of life and consciousness within them. Life is not to be looked upon as something which is defined in a very limited way. Life exists in all things.... You must realize that there is a higher science. This is a spiritual science that understands and encompasses all natural laws and that explains the delicate relationships that exist between them.

Appendix G

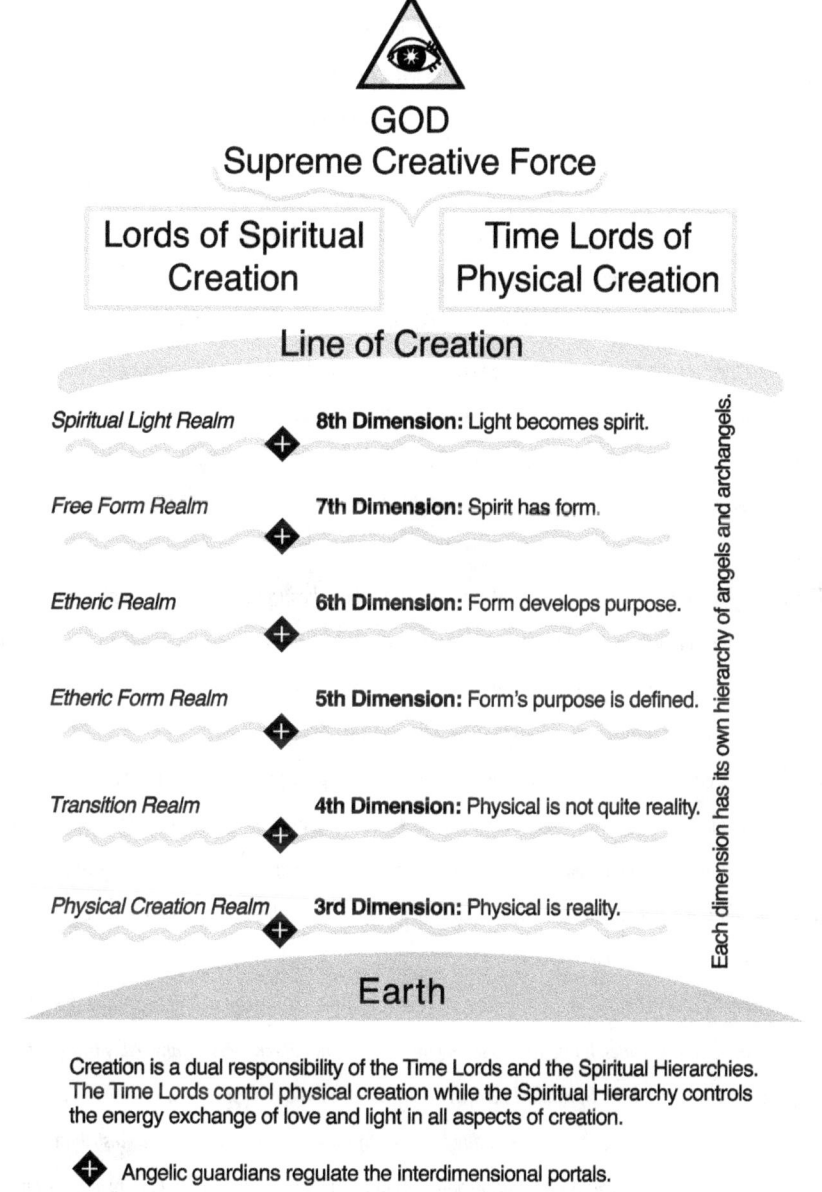

Figure 20: Dimensions of Physical Creation[7]

---

[7] Essene, You Are Becoming 143.

These spiritual sciences contain the laws of guardianship. They state that first and foremost a guardian is one who brings in the energies of creation (spiritual light and love) and regulates them for the planetary life sphere or biosphere, as it is known to modern science. At present on planet Earth there exist two major species that are designated as guardian groups. *The first such species called a cetacean (the whales and the dolphins) who now form the basic guardianship of the planet. The second designated guardians are the Earth human species originally brought from other star systems to their present location on planet Earth.* (142-145)

…What is needed now is for Earth humans to understand what a guardian is and the important mission that guardians share with their Spiritual Hierarchy. You might well be wondering what guardianship's basic components are—or in Earth terms what your job description as a guardian requires.

Guardianship can best be described by observing the energies of the cetaceans. Through the use of their rituals, their sonar songs and their travels, they vivify the biosphere. Whale song has been found throughout all oceans of the world. It is also found in, and resonates throughout, the skies of the Earth. It exists even in the deepest parts of Africa, the Americas, Asia, and Europe. Because the energies of the cetaceans can be found both in the sky and in the water, those great energies they bring forth in their song create the resonance that sustains life. Indeed, their rituals have brought forth ongoing and glorious regenesis of life.

Every year from February through August, cetaceans from both hemispheres perform rituals of song that make possible the opening of windows in this biosphere for the energies needed for the reproduction of all species. This procreative act produces the new children of all species and makes possible the continuation of life on Earth. These rituals empower the continuation of the vast multitude of life forms that are a unique aspect of your planet.

Furthermore, guardianship also means stewardship. This concept requires that the guardians must set forth energies that not only provide for the renewal of species on the planet, but also give those species an understanding of what it is that they are accomplishing (a gradual growth toward consciousness). This stewardship means that they must either sacrifice the creative energies that they hold in themselves, or else use their psychic and other full consciousness energies to accommodate procreation and the sustaining of life on the planet.

Stewardship is a very unique and important process. It is more than shepherding the many species of your planet through their day-to-day activities. It also means setting up maintenance life energies by physically transmuting the creative energies given daily by the Earth's Spiritual Hierarchy. This action allows each species of your world to maintain itself. It also means that the energies being received every day from the Spiritual Hierarchy have to be distributed across the entire biosphere. Guardians must consciously and subconsciously maintain these energies so that they are dispersed in a proper and correct manner. This whole process is done every day by the cetaceans. They also consciously realize the power of this process of interdimensional energy exchange.

Guardianship, therefore, contributes to and preserves the role of Lady Gaia. It allows planet Earth—along with its life forms—to sustain themselves and to do so with a flourish of abundance. On your planet, all species have attained an unbelievable variety and have thrived in all environments that exist. Yet humans who are the third and final part of this triangle (humans, cetaceans, and Spiritual Hierarchy) have totally forgotten, and therefore completely ignored, the important aspects of stewardship that they must now thoroughly understand and begin to follow.

At this time, let us suggest that a good steward knows and understands his flock. He or she does his or her shepherding in a way that teaches the members of the flock to comprehend and ascertain what it takes to maintain themselves and to flourish. Stewardship by humans should be one which recognizes and protects the Earth's environment because the environment—like the one surrounding a shepherd's flock, is the one that sustains all life.

You must learn that the Earth's environment is the foundation of your physical existence, not something to be conquered or abused. Truly, your planetary environment must be understood, for that very environment that supports you humans with important life-giving energies, must in turn be sustained with transmuted energies from you. This knowledge of your reciprocal roles is the first important part of guardianship. The good steward practices it and you as stewards of the Earth must learn it....

... [C]oncepts of love and light—given through consciousness to all living beings—form the basis for beginning to understand how to be good Earth stewards, as well as shepherds, for your own species. (145-147)

So far we have described the environmental aspect as well as the spiritual aspect of guardianship, but there is a third component that we have not yet discussed. This aspect requires your recognition that other guardian species exist on your planet, and that you must interact with them in a way that shows your appreciation and love for what they do.... Earth humans have failed... to understand that guardianship is indeed shared. You must learn to share with your cetacean brothers and sisters in ways that allow them, as well as yourselves, to interact through love and high consciousness with each other....

... You have come to Earth to implement the Spiritual Hierarchy's instructions, not to ignore your role and the role of other guardians who are on your world. Remember, there exists on Earth a great and incredible abundance and this abundance will beget even greater abundance if it is properly attended to. This rationale is what we wish to have all people on your planet understand.

We galactic humans are a guardian species; therefore, so are Earth humans, though you may have temporarily forgotten. The Spiritual Hierarchy of angelic beings that surrounds you now is helping you achieve higher consciousness and will aid you in this process. Thus, look away from your upside-down civilization and analyze what needs fixing. This process of fixing is one that is quite simple—and humans are good "fixers." (147-148)

Washta: What is happening on your planet right now is that every human, whether fully conscious or not, is undergoing a great degree of genetic alteration. These alterations are preparing humans for the stupendous transformation process and the ascension that will occur in the next few years.

Consequently, humans have experienced a great deal of what they have thought to be physical ailments—ailments or difficulties that are, in fact, simple alterations in brain cell patterning, disruption of the nervous system circuits, alterations of the heart, or genetic alterations of cellular structure. That is why many sudden and unexplained conditions, diseases or illnesses have occurred and then left very quickly after they came. This is how you can know that the changes that are about to occur on your planet are on course. Part of the process being brought in by the Spiritual Hierarchy now is to lengthen some of these processes, but at the same time to speed up the karmic dissolution that is now occurring on your planet.

A brief slowdown was recently advised by the Spiritual Hierarchy, because they felt that many humans on planet Earth were panicking at the changes that were occurring around them. This slowdown does not mean any major decrease will persist; it is just a temporary adjustment, like slowing down from 80 miles per hour to 75 miles per hour. We and you are still moving at great speed so that the divine plan can be achieved! In our scannings and evaluations of the human body, we find that it is holding up to this energy acceleration. (157-158)

So let us summarize that which is essential to remember and practice. Guardianship works through the eight dimensions of creation. It spreads itself through the great Spiritual Hierarchies and permeates down to your world. Around the Spiritual Hierarchy is manifested the physical universe that you are a part of. As a guardian species, galactic humans are a being of light, a spiritual as well as physical being. Your capability to be spirit-in-matter is what makes you a unique creation. In addition, you have been given a special consciousness that extends beyond the mere reflexes of life such as sex, hunger, thirst, and dying. You go beyond the mere physicalness of all of this. You are a being who has been put upon a planet as a responsible overseer or steward of other life. This happens because you are capable of full consciousness.

The cetaceans who exist around you are an example of what this full consciousness implies in everyday living. When you look at their guardianship, you will see that they have unselfishly and totally committed their lives to the process of bringing forth those energies that allow your planetary system to evolve and to survive. This activity is what Earth humans have not done. (148-149)

We have said that Earth's physical structure was created for a divine purpose. This divine purpose was established by the angelics under the great Godhead that was moved through the heart of God into reality. It was done for one purpose—to bring forth a creation of physical light. All Earth humans must understand this process and assume their awakening role.

What is about to happen to your planet and your solar system... will erase your ignorance and allow all of you to fully understand what guardianship is. Guardianship, as we continue to state, is a process of creative **stewardship and stewardship is a means to bring full consciousness to bear in the actions and activities of one species as it affects another.** For you humans sit at the top of a huge chain of life and this chain of life does not merely consist of animals and plants. As mentioned, it also includes rocks, soil, water, sky, and everything that creeps or crawls. Your Christian Bible is quite explicit about your place in the dominion role!

Remember, also, that there are energy devas in created things who act together to create the great cycle of life in you and in all living things around you. This cycle of life is the key that lies at the heart of everything that is happening on your planet. Earth humans must understand this process and be fully prepared to accept and practice their reasons for being on Earth. You are present as part of a great triangle of consciousness—Cetacean, Earth human, and Lady Gaia—all who work together to create a life sphere of elegance and of light that brings your planet's energies into focus as an exquisite showcase for all to see.

You must not look at planets as merely being 3rd-dimensional objects which orbit around a particular star until the time comes when the death of that star brings a planet's life to an end. This action is not the process to be examined. All things in the universe exist for a specific purpose. This particular purpose is one that you must understand and apply if you wish to advance in your consciousness and future galactic roles—even universal ones.

Therefore, remember you are a guardian of light, of love, and of consciousness; and you are a part of this great guardianship triangle of humans, cetaceans and Spiritual Hierarchy. Your planet is now on the verge of a new Golden Age that will lead to a rejuvenation and a welcoming home of Earth humans. It comes so you can be the galactic creation that God intended! In this discovery, you will coexist in a fantastic relationship with your extraordinary planet, and with other guardians species like the cetaceans. In these relationships you will also work hand-in-hand with that shining group of angels and ascended masters called the Spiritual Hierarchy of God. This partnership will ignite your hearts with love and fill your eternity with joy, wherever you may advance. (149-150)

galactic human civilization

... [Next] let us begin ... [to discuss] the history and origins of human civilization.

The very first human civilizations were established in the star system of Vega, the brightest star in the Lyra constellation, some six million years ago. During this time, Vega's human inhabitants developed the primary rudiments of a truly interplanetary culture. *This culture was based on two main principles that were delivered as the four primary laws of society.*

The first of these two principles was the importance of the personal growth of the individual. The civilization's foundation belief was that an individual's growth in consciousness could develop only by fully exploring one's higher soul as well as concurrently giving service to others. Love was seen by them as the ability to thoroughly understand another soul force and then to use that knowledge to better understand oneself.

The second principle stated that each person's soul light shines on everyone in a unique way. Each soul light contains a piece of the great puzzle that composes the united human family. It was the duty of one's friends and family to help bring this light into its full and complete brightness. Let us briefly review galactic civilization and discuss its underlying principles and laws of society in greater detail.

The origins of galactic civilization evolved from what are called the galactic and interdimensional Spiritual Hierarchies. These spiritual lords of time and space established within their realms (galaxies and star systems) a distinct series of unique physical presences. This enterprise was done because planets, stars and other energy forms needed a complementary physical guardian to aid them in establishing the white light of creation throughout the physical universe. To this end, the Spiritual Hierarchies created special life forms (various humans and nonhumans of high sentience). These life forms were established as part of a guardianship that would act with the Spiritual Hierarchies to enable the energies of creation to operate at maximum efficiency through physical creation.

This concept of planetary and star system stewardship is what is called the guardian nature of all human culture. It is the foundation upon which all humans have formed their fully conscious civilizations. As Earth humans grow in awareness and increase their consciousness, it is natural for the environmental movement and the stewardship of the Earth to gain support and grow in importance. Therefore, it is essential to learn how these processes of caretaking and guardianship are related to the growth of human consciousness. Learning about this guardianship process will enable Earth humans to better understand how to successfully create a galactic culture here on your planet, for the Lyran culture is part of Sirius and you of Earth are now under an increasing Sirian influence.

This guardian nature that the Spiritual Hierarchy originally gave to all humans is a great gift, for it was based on a democratic system of social laws with four explicit aspects (See Figure 21: Four Basic Social Laws.) These four laws can be used by human civilization to conduct itself in full accordance with the Spiritual Hierarchies. They also enable every human to reach full consciousness, thereby achieving full service for themselves and especially to each other. In applying these laws, Earth humans will earn their place in the great galactic guardianship plan for the entire human species. And they will bring human civilization to its fullest possible flowering. Accordingly, let us consider these four laws to see exactly what they represent. (159-160)

To aid all beings who incarnate into the Syrian realm of full human consciousness, each clan provides to its members a series of counselors who are attached to each clan's temple system. These clan temples, located among and upon the major planetary grid points, serve as the core for the web of consciousness that exists throughout the planet. Here, meditations and exercises are given that permit you to successfully pass through the various life crises you could encounter while acknowledging your personal growth in consciousness through the Law of the One and the Law of the Two. It is in the clan temple that the first concepts of being a planetary guardian are established. . . .

As one went through life from early childhood to more mature adulthood, one encountered a specific set of lessons and rituals. These rituals and lessons would help beings to understand why they came into physical life, and the purpose for which they incarnated into this physical world. Each being believed he/she had a sacred reason for existence—a specific gift—that would aid not only self, but also the group, the civilization, the planet, and star system—the whole of existence. It was the intent of one's counselor to aid in determining these essential designs. By so doing, the counseling process would allow the individual to fully explore his or her own inner selfhood, as well as those responsibilities that were fundamental to this growth.

Rituals or rites to us are simply the accomplishment of something or the doing of a certain task. Rituals on your planet usually are meant as some long lethargic ceremony in which somebody speaks extensively and everyone falls asleep. This is not what we do! An example of a ritual for a child would be to take the child to the beach and have it just play with the sand

and the rocks, feel the energy of the devas around it, and thereby understand the purpose and correlation of this soil and rock to the great energy patterns of the planet, itself. Thus the child understands its own physicalness and feels its relationship with all physical things, as well. As the child grows many of these little rituals are performed. (162-164)

... [So,] education in the Lyran/Sirian tradition was done for two reasons. First, education prepared an individual for a specific life task. This project was to assist beings in understanding how this service would express love and personal growth. Secondly, it was also believed that all individuals had to learn who they were—and so education encompassed this aspect as

---

Four Basic Social Laws ...

Law of the One:
The goal of every being is to discover their soul path for personal growth and service.

Law of the Two:
The power of creation can be utilized through loving closeness with another being. This close relationship with, and caring for one another, leads to a deeper knowledge of guardianship.

Law of the Three:
The bonding created by one's close relationship with self, friends, family and clan develops the web of global or planetary interdependency.

Law of the Four:
The Law of the Four is the Law of the Three expanded to larger groups such as clan-to-clan and planetary-to-solar (star) system.

Figure 21: Four Basic Social Laws[8]

well. The Lyrans believed that knowing oneself would lead one to originate those services that would create the interconnected web of consciousness and light. Each individual was consequently taught to remember the memories of other lifetimes and realities. These memories were not to be forgotten, but rather were to be enhanced during the course of each lifetime. Life in the Lyran/Sirian tradition was not a brief series of unconnected incidents. Rather, it was comprised of a series of conscious realities that prepared each soul force for its eventual return to the higher life energies that originally created it. **This great love**

---

[8] Essene, You Are Becoming 161.

of the universe and its cyclic order was the foundation of the Lyran civilization's cosmic plan and sustained its successful completion.

The Time Lords further stipulated that these laws could be extended outside of an immediate star system by creating an expanding system of laws in which the Law of the One was changed into the Law of the Four, and then enlarged through these next four laws to the Law of the Five, Six, and Seven.... By the time one reached the Law of the Seven, the Law of the Four had been increased to a planetary and solar **Kha'Baa** (group soul force) that could be evolved into an eventual **Khas'Koo** for an entire star sector. Galactic humans could thus pass on to their offspring the sacred laws governing society as created by the Time Lords and embodied in the divine energies of the One, the Four, the Seven and the Ten.

Every individual learned that the key to devotion and inner reflection of the soul force energy was within the instructions given by the clan counselors. These counselors were highly respected members of their clan. Their inner growth and high soul force qualified them to give instruction in the sacred task of leading others into higher states of consciousness. Counselors also knew prescribed rituals and specific meditations that could be given to those whom they counseled. In this way, the culture continued from childhood to adulthood and ritual was an essential aspect of personal development. These rituals helped each individual to understand the nature of the multidimensional universe and establish a relationship to it as a growing and fully conscious being. This essence of selfhood merged with a need for service to others and to the Time Lord's ultimate creation—the physical universe.

Each individual was taught, then, that one incarnated into the physical universe in order to fulfill a specific purpose. Also, each individual was taught from birth that memories from other life times must not be forgotten. Thus, special counselors were assigned to each newborn and to their parents to begin the process of keeping the past life memories alive and the new life goals in perspective.

It was believed by those in the Lyran/Sirian culture that the life process of birth should have a special set of meditations and rituals to welcome the newborn into the community and identify its specific purpose—its reason for the newly acquired physical reality. Birth was, therefore, the beginning of a joyous lifelong gift into the great web of consciousness that surrounded each and every individual.

Under the Law of the One, every individual had to discover its own life and love center and learn how to use this life and love center to appreciate its purposes for physical selfhood. This duty began at birth with the aforementioned rituals and was maintained throughout early childhood. Parents in this tradition were properly prepared and aided by the assigned clan counselors. Each pregnancy began with a system of preparation for the newborn and its needs. To parent in a Lyran/Sirian culture was a great privilege, intended to foster and witness the beginning of the never-ending cycle of life.

Life's purposes and its joys were shared not only by the immediate family, but also by the clan structure. Love was an important part of the consciousness of each individual and became a vital aspect of each individual's life. For example, as one passed through childhood, one quickly learned about his or her origins and initial purposes. A young child was encouraged to discover the joy of play as well as the mutual importance of each other's selfhood to the conscious web of life surrounding them. Children learned that humans are a guardian species created for the purpose of aiding the universal Spiritual Hierarchies of light and love, and of bringing order and light to the physical universe. This responsibility is one all humans must take seriously. Each individual, from earliest childhood, was taught to act as a guardian or steward of planets and stars. This was a sacred task.

Guardianship responsibilities were made known by each counselor to every young child, and lessons about guardianship were constantly learned by ritual example. For example, a key part of learning about guardianship was a daily meditation ritual performed upon arising from a brief mid-morning nap. All humans were required to perform this ritual in order to maintain the biosphere. These rituals were designed for all ages and were learned as a preparation for adult life. Young individuals also learned by exploring rites taught to them as a kind of play. It was common for counselors to take young children to the clan temples and to allow them to participate in the daily ceremonies to enhance the planetary life force energies. In discovering the significance of this daily ritual to human civilization, children discerned the various levels of spiritual energies that surround the physical creation. This ritual helped a child or a young adult to learn about the Time Lords, the Spiritual Hierarchies and the child's role in the ever-evolving process of creation. It was a vital link between human selfhood and the constant re-creation of the physical universe that surrounded all humans.

It is an important part of the laws of galactic society that all children become aware of the many worlds that surround them. By the end of early childhood, a child is able to relate inner purposes to present life and present purpose to past life activities. The continuity of the life cycle is fully explained to the children. The life cycle is not to be discontinuous nor is the purpose of each past life to be completely forgotten. Life is a continual process from which guardianship evolves as a vital part. The self is not seen as a disjointed or alienated ego, but as the connected part of a web of consciousness. Thus, ritual assists the young child as well as the adult to understand his or her life plan and to express the specific role that the guardian spirits have deemed applicable for this lifetime.

It is important that those family members and friends who constitute a child's physical reality be included in everyday activities and ritual. Every individual chooses both parents and responsibilities for certain reasons. These reasons must be explored and understood by everyone involved in the creation of a child's physical reality. The key focus at all times is not only to encourage the development of selfhood, but also to develop an exploration of those connections that are part of creating this selfhood. Important ritual practices (directed play) are instituted during childhood to help the child understand the role of nurturing life and how that role relates to discovering his selfhood—such as playing with small animals and appreciating their role in the biosphere. It is necessary that the guardian role of each human be discovered for it is a process that runs deep in the soul force.

Each life cycle is an opportunity to explore new realities and to determine how one will eventually fit into the vast web of light that is human consciousness. This network of light encompasses all other sentient species and allows the human soul force to eventually merge with others to form a great galactic web of light as prophesied by the Time Lords. These relationships between species and the more important individual relationships between human civilizations, are based upon the relationships of the Law of the Two. Relationships of closeness bring a full understanding of what it is to serve another through love. This love energy is the basis for human civilization and the major reason for its continuing existence.

To summarize, these laws—the Laws of the One, the Four, the Seven and the Ten—are to be given to your civilization when the mass landings occur in the period just before the arrival of the photon belt. This is because your civilization is to become a civilization of fully conscious galactic humans. Once you enter into the web of galactic consciousness, you must know the rules and accept the responsibilities required to successfully have your guardianship succeed in the solar system. Humans who dwell upon Earth are about to be transformed. You must be prepared for all that is about to happen. That is why this Sirian Council has just given you a basic primer on Sirian law. These laws of relationship are vital; yet you must understand that these laws constitute only a mere beginning. This simple introduction is for you to explore and probe so that you may get a better understanding of the full meaning of Lyran/Sirian (galactic human) civilization—your very own heritage! (165-169)

[the original galactic creation myth]

Washta: The original galactic creation myth is about 50 million years old for physical sentient beings but older still for many non-human species. Some of these non-human species have returned to the etheric light form. More recently, about six million years ago in the Lyran constellation—specifically in the Vega star system—humans were given sentience and rudiments of civilization.

This creation myth, given for the human species, stated that there would be 100 light-star demonstration systems created. Your solar system—which we call Solis, meaning "Great Light" — was the closest of these 100 demonstration star systems to us on Sirius. You present the potential manifestation of a glorious showcase experiment bringing light into darkness.

Basically, our creation myth begins in a similar way to many of the Earth myths contained in your religious texts and guides, such as the Bible and in many texts found in India. The various basic texts of Hinduism are the oldest unpurged works that contain a similarity to the original galactic human creation myth, so let us begin with that.

The original galactic human creation myth says that in the beginning there was the great darkness. The darkness was there because the Creator had decided to make this creation one in which there would be light coming out of the darkness, so God assigned the Time Lords to accomplish this feat. And lo, over many incredible eons, the great pulse of time was created by the Time Lords. Then with the power of the Supreme Creative Force, time pulsed into the darkness and there was a great light in the darkness, from which came many things.

One of these creations was the birth of all the stars and galaxies, for they were the great lights hung in the darkness. At the same time, however, darkness had also created its own dark light as part of God's original creation plan. So even darkness would have light that would later be transmuted into the great holy white light that the Time Lords had brought down.

And so both light and darkness were part of the one creation in the beginning—each of which was allowed to create its own dimensions and levels. This brought forth duality and various kinds of spiritual energies that made everything around us possible. Then out of this duality there arose both light and dark celestial beings and these beings became a prototype for the many species created of both light and dark.

Appendix G

The light forces now created many species, one of which was a great primate from the Vega system. From the Vegan creation came the energies that brought forth what is today called "human," and the energies of the celestial hosts allowed this human to develop and to spread across the galaxy much as other creations of light had done. (194-195)

[*why our solar system was important*]

Virginia: ... Could you clarify why our Solar system was important? It sounds like we were out on the galactic fringes, but you say there was an important spiritual energy here?

Washta: Your solar system was chosen among the one hundred others previously mentioned, to bring in the first human prototype energies from Vega. Then of that one hundred which were chosen, planet Earth and your solar system were given the first great etheric civilization of any kind. That is why your planet and its host, the Spiritual Hierarchy, are considered to have a special blessed position. This explains why, when humans were forced to withdraw from Earth, they spread out across this sector of the galaxy. But they made a pledge to re-enter your solar system and bring human civilization back to it once again. This was part of their pledge, then, to complete the karma of humans in the Vega system and reclaim this system for the light —as required by the Vegan and Earth Spiritual Hierarchies.

However, the histories of the past few million years have not accomplished this great pledge. In the beginning there was success, but as we have already explained the last 10,000 years on Earth have been disastrous. This misfortune began approximately 25,000 years ago when the Lemurians were destroyed by the Atlanteans, as we have previously mentioned.

It is unfortunate that the dark energy perceived the value of Earth's place in the creation myth, for that is why the dark forces came here to Solis, your solar system. And that is why your planet continues to have such an important position in the balance of power even though its Sun sits in a minor position in this section of our galaxy.

Virginia: ... Earth was one of that special 100 human light-star systems. What happened to the other 99 light-star systems?

Washta: Of those other 99, only 90 were able to maintain their energy patterns and most of them developed non-human civilizations. Many of them in the Orion system, for example, brought forth some very advanced amphibious groups that are incredibly spiritual. They are, in fact, mostly etheric in form. They look quite different from what a human might expect, yet their energies and their love are so great that when any human encounters them, all apprehensions are immediately transmuted by their loving vibration. Many times the dinoid and reptoid civilizations of Orion have attempted to conquer the amphibian group's star systems only to fail. The amphibiod spiritual energies of these great civilizations was so highly developed that they were invisible to the reptoid or the dinoid invasions. At a deeper level, these invasions could not succeed because the darker energies did not wish to be enlightened at that time.(195-196)

[*the galactic federation*]

[**Washta:**] To further aid you in understanding the value of group consciousness and group energy as it relates to the multidimensional nature of the spiritual and creative energy of the physical universe, you may wish to study galactic time and discover how it relates to the continuing creation of the physical universe (197).

> ... [G]alactic time can have [a profound influence] in your everyday lives, but can you dare imagine its value to a group of highly-focused people? Let us review a few simple facts about what the Mayan Calendar is all about, for both individuals and groups. Please remember that your present 365-day Earth calendar is not a spiritual one but a material world calendar using physical, linear thinking. It is spiritually unconscious, so to say, and does not clarify or identify the vibrations which our galactic time contains and which we use to maintain and advance spiritual growth on many levels.
>
> **Time is the initiator pulse that makes all things in physical reality possible.** It is stated in an ancient Sirian proverb about physical creation that the Time Lords were handed the great pulse of time by the Supreme Creator Force.
>
> So let us examine this great pulse of creation—time—as a way of understanding and experiencing reality. In our galactic civilizations, we use Time Keepers to keep us informed about the actions of the Time Lords. Time Keepers are persons who dedicate themselves to understanding the underlying meanings of the universal pulse of time and to communicate with the Spiritual Hierarchy and the Time Lords on how physical creation is evolving. In other words, they could be compared favorably to the oracles of ancient Greece, Rome, and Egypt on your planet. To further emphasize this important point to Earth humans, we must ask that you look at the Mayan civilization of MesoAmerica which was given a sacred galactic calendar by selected elements of Pleiadean and Arcturian Time Keepers at the beginning of the Mayan classical period (4th century AD through the 9th century AD).
>
> This sacred galactic calendar has 20 Mayan glyphs. Their corresponding four harmonics and the 13 tones of creation were superimposed by the Mayan Time Keepers to conceive what was called a ***K'in***. These 13 tones are used to make possible an experiential logic that signifies the best way to experience a particular day. These day patterns are mirrored daily in the sacred 260-day calendar of life called the ***Tzolkin*** (pronounced zoulkin). This 260-day cycle is sacred, indeed.
>
> As just stated, in this sacred calendar, the 20 glyphs are combined with the 13 tones of creation to create what is called a ***K'in*** or experiential logic of the day. Each Mayan glyph encompasses all of the 13 tones of creation to form each one of the 260 ***K'in***. The 13 tones of creation are unity, challenge, activation, definition, radiance, equality, attunement, integrity, intention, manifestation, liberation, cooperation, and transcendence.
>
> If you knew which influences were being energized every day, as we do, you would cooperate with that reality and the powerful manifesting energies of Creation, instead of pushing your own uniformed intentions and attempting activities at the wrong time or in a non-productive sequence of manifestation.
>
> There are some Earth teachers who understand and can explain this galactic time material to you.... We highly recommend this topic,... [with] its many essential characteristics and qualities. Just remember your Earth time is vanishing and galactic time will eventually replace it. (200-201)
>
> We of the Sirian Council... wish to describe something about our own history as galactic humans and also about the organization called the Galactic Federation that Earth will soon be entering as a new member.

Appendix G

  The Galactic Federation was formed about 4.5 million years ago to prevent interdimensional dark forces from dominating and exploiting this galaxy. This interdimensional dark force had seeded the Milky Way Galaxy with its own kind of computer-like, cold-hearted beings. Their appearance was mainly in the form of a reptoid or a dinoid individual as described earlier. These dark beings spread across the galaxy and began to successfully conquer thousands of star systems. These reptoids/dinoids, however, eventually reached an area of the galaxy where free-willed sentient human beings had created several galactic civilizations which were their technological match.

  What followed, about four million years ago, was a period of brief but very barbaric stellar wars which were quickly interspersed by periods of peace. To a limited extent, this war and peace pattern has continued even into present times. As the attacks continued across the galaxy, those of us who were the enemies of this Dinoid/Reptoid Alliance became more organized. We saw the need to develop a highly diversified and effective organization that could act as an umbrella for both the coordination of the galaxy's defenses, and also as a forum that would permit necessary human and nonhuman cultural and governmental exchanges.

  The Galactic Federation sees itself as a sort of United Nations of star systems whose sole purpose is to create an organization that will allow light to continue to flow into our Milky Way galaxy. At present there are over 100,000 star systems and star leagues in the Galactic Federation, and recent additions between 1988 and 1993 have increased membership to almost 200,000 members. The primary basis of this galactic light of Creation is love. (203-204)

  Since the Galactic Federation considers itself an organization of fully conscious and peaceful civilizations, it is constantly on the lookout for acceptable civilizations that meet its criteria for membership. When any planet or a series of planets in any star system reaches prescribed levels of technological and cultural development, these civilizations are contacted after a thorough scientific evaluation. This scientific evaluation covers an extremely broad spectrum of cultural, scientific, and spiritual qualifications.

  Your planet and surrounding solar system have been given a dispensation from Galactic Federation rules on membership because of the effects of the Sirian Governing Council and your Spiritual Hierarchy. The Spiritual Hierarchy reminded all Galactic Federation Councils of the special position of your solar system as both an important showcase solar system and as the underriding cause for human sentiency in the first place. This argument finally overturned the karmic laws established by Pleiadean control of your solar system since the fall of Atlantis some 10,000 years ago, and permitted the granting of **full membership to Earth in the Galactic Federation on March 5, 1993 Earth time.** (204)

  …As mentioned, the main purpose of the Galactic Federation is to hasten the creation of highly sentient light-oriented galactic civilizations across our galaxy. This purpose is divided into three main parts: first, the space mission;[9] second, the liaison groups;[10] and third, the interdivisional forums… [comprised of] the various Galactic Federation Regional and Local Federation Governing Councils (205).

  The Galactic Federation is not here to exploit Earth humans. Rather, it is here to promote them into higher consciousness and to save a beleaguered planet. We are here to help birth a new human spirit and advance the entire human race into *their intended true role as a guardian species once again. In this increased consciousness, Earth humans will then reclaim their relationship with other galactic humans spread all across the galaxy (212).*

... [Toward this end] policy change began to take effect in the late 1980s. It has allowed Sirians to alter the Sun's polarity and to research the methods for the first emergence of the ascension process [and] to evaluate [your] biosphere in a new way—a way that would allow your solar system to be altered back to what it was at the time of Lemuria (213).

Virginia: *... Could you discuss whether there has even been on this planet, since Lemuria, any nation or government that even approaches the application of Lemurian ideals?*

Washta: *There exists, not on the surface of your planet but underground, since the end of Lemurian times (25,000 years ago), what is called in your mythologies the kingdom of Agartha or Shamballa. It has become a huge underground network connecting all major continents to the capital which exists beneath what is today called the nation of Tibet. This civilization has remained in various below-surface enclaves around the planet, being one with the Spiritual Hierarchies to bring humans into higher consciousness. They will again unite with surface humans once the mission of bringing full consciousness to your planet has been completed. (220)*

Washta: *The most important concept for Earth humanity to know about universes at the present time is that a shift is occurring. If we may call the universes "dimensions," there is a shift occurring from the third to the fifth dimension. This has a major effect. And it also has affected all other dimensions or universes up to the seventh dimension. Thus we have roughly five of these that are being affected from the third through the seventh dimension. This is because the increases in consciousness on your planet have required that the Spiritual Hierarchy make many dimensional shifts. As they now adjust the interdimensional energy exchanges, your planet can be prepared for movement into its new full consciousness.*

Virginia: *So are you really indicating that we would be better off—rather than using the word 'universe' as a physical place—to think of a universe as a dimension of awareness or consciousness?*

Washta: *That is what we would prefer because dimensions, once they rise above the so-called fourth and fifth dimension, become fully spiritual. Therefore, they do not exist in any concept similar to the so-called third-dimensional physical framework that everyone on your planet considers to be the basic aspect of their reality. (220-221)*

Virginia: *So where does that leave Sirians as human beings who have full consciousness?*

Washta: *We are fully conscious beings existing in this third dimension, but because of this fully conscious capability we can also commune with the angelic forces of other dimensions. We are thus a true guardian species because the Spiritual*

---

[9] Divided into science and exploration teams and forces for the protection of these teams (Essene, You Are Becoming 205-207).

[10] The liaison groups are comprised of over two billion communication networkers acting as a central unit of sorts and providing the necessary information to all divisions of the Galactic Federation so that they may make wise decisions (Essene, You Are Becoming 207).

Appendix G

Hierarchies that control the energies of this dimension, as well as the creation hierarchies of the Time Lords, are able to speak to us, and we are able to interact with them, too. This communication occurs on your planet in only rare individuals, whereas for us it is the usual experience of our entire civilization and an aspect of the reality we actually utilize.

Virginia: So in other words, a Sirian is a third-dimensional physical being with fourth- and/or fifth-dimensional awareness.

Washta: We have interdimensional capabilities because we are able to completely transform our physical third-dimensional type of body to a light-body that allows us to move around in other aspects of reality.

Virginia: Then your species is not totally, physically solid?

Washta: Earth humans and Sirians are very similar. If you were to see me walk down the street you could easily bump right into me, or converse with me just as you could with any other human on your planet. We are both physical beings, but Sirian humans also have the capability, because we are in complete control of our physicality, to transform our bodies into an interdimensional light-body or even to increase its usual frequency where the average Earth human would think it had disappeared. (221)

Washta: We believe that the coming century, or roughly the next 100 years or less of Earth calendar time, will successfully bring the end to warring and violence. We believe that we are approaching not only a millennium of great change in your solar system, but we are also achieving the great ascension of light in this galaxy after battling the darkness for eons. This is because of the phenomenal and unbelievable shift in consciousness by the dark energy forces toward the light. At present, over half of the galaxy has moved into the light, whereas at the beginning of the 1980s that figure was less than a quarter of the galactic population. If this change continues at this pace, we estimate that by the end of the next century the entire galaxy will be able to ascend. This positive shift is also being reported by many other galaxies with whom we are now in communication. Their observations agree with ours, even down to the time estimates. We are therefore all the more confident about our approaching galactic enlightenment.

Virginia: How many galaxies does the Galactic Federation negotiate with at this time?

Washta: We are negotiating with approximately 50 galaxies and already have two of these galaxies as members. It is our deep hope that in the next few decades we can make as many new intergalactic connections as those we are now forming with our own galactic family. To us, this is a great omen that an amazing change is going on in our galaxy and that the time of the great myth of the light (the divine prophecy)—a basic foundation belief of all that the Galactic Federation works toward—is about to occur. (223)

Washta: … we have visited two planetary systems in Pegasus that are not in your present category as a showcase solar system but are very primitive. …

Our experiences have also included sharing our patterns of curing illness or providing food and resources for beings in need. On your planet, though, we have found the beings to be extremely rebellious and very much into their own concept of free will. This has caused us to observe them cautiously and has created many great difficulties in interacting with some humans on your planet. However, we consider this to be part of bringing light to your planet. As a showcase planet, it is one that will bring full consciousness of free will use and end all concepts and behaviors which are not based upon divine principles....

... There will still be a degree of rebelliousness as energy shifts occur because many human children are taught erroneous concepts and have become adjusted to that backward concept of civilization that Earth presently holds. However, we have been told and have seen by scanning humans on the planet, that beneath this shell of rebelliousness there sits a great angelic light. Once full consciousness is restored to the human physical body, this light will more easily combine with the body and produce the effects that we predict will form a new galactic civilization.

Earth humans will have a new concept of working in a full-consciousness civilization with free will on a third-dimensional level. Earth humans are the ones destined to create the great mastery of the third dimension that many of us have come close to, but which your solar system and your planet will actually achieve. That is why Earth is destined to be a great and glorious showcase once again, thereby fulfilling the divine prophecy of eons past....

... A full gamut of darkness has been delivered to your planet, as well as one of light. Now, however, your planet will combine both to produce its own unique civilization—one that will act as a showcase. Therefore, we know that even though you are but children barely entering primary school, to use an analogy, you will rapidly be the PhDs who will teach many of this galaxy's civilizations great lessons that all galactic civilizations must also learn....

... [T]he Spiritual Hierarchy has, so to speak, set up the soul contracts and the ways that it would be done. The Spiritual Hierarchy has excellently planned and organized the structure of what is now happening. The principles and the agreements that they have reached with all human souls on your planet make possible the great changes that are about to occur.

Before all human souls were allowed to incarnate on your planet, they were told that they would have to formally agree under the precepts of the divine plan and divine right order to the following two principles. First, they agreed to allow the Spiritual Hierarchy to determine when a divine intervention (to restore full consciousness) would be necessary and how it would occur. Second, they agreed to act as true Earth guardians (after the divine intervention) when the Spiritual Hierarchy so decreed. (224-225)

[from "Virginia's afterword"]

... Literally everything that is received from any source must, I believe, be held in the arena of potentiality as it is cross-checked with other guidance....

I am finding that no one source or teacher is working totally alone in this time of group consciousness—rather each contributes a unique portion of their talent to this enormously simple but also quite complex human experience. Our purest intuitives are surely sharing a quality of energy that can lead us through various challenges at the absolutely highest level of our combined emotional stability and innate wisdom. Since everything is energy, we must ourselves seek its highest vibratory frequency to fully experience the loving assistance that the divine has promised us, and is now delivering. I believe it will require our devoted attention to achieve this energy's purpose and direction within our personal lives, our group relationships, and our *global responsibilities, not to mention galactic endeavors. We now need each other more than ever before, during this ascension [shift] with its enormous variations, potentials and levels of awareness.*

… Our bonded love and willingness to serve the highest god will guide and protect us as we spiral through the dimensional information barriers and interdimensional openings of truth.

There will be new vocabularies to deal with and our actual spiritual experience may be grander than what our limited language references to terms such as gates, star gates, portals and frequency bands can define and explain…. [B]ut it is love that will guide us, more than we can even imagine, at this stage of our awareness. (229-230)

*Appendix H: Recollections from a Guided **Corridor** Meditation*[1]

The **corridor** is all white — about twenty feet across and some fifty or sixty feet in length or more.[2] There's a feeling of great wholeness, refinement and grace about it — not punctuated by windows — just a long and not too narrow expanse of roomness, decidedly not of hallway or typical corridor proportions or dimensions but not of a warehouse breadth or lateral boundarylessness either — wonderfully high ceilings yet not calling attention to themselves as might have been the case had the room been far narrower. And flat ceilings so that ceilingness didn't call further attention to itself either, as it would have if sloped or pitched or vaulted. The whole expanse of twenty by sixty feet or more of floor is paved in seamless marble — a white marble — a fairytale blend created in the ethers of the creamed viscosity of that sparkle-free white between the veins of grey in Yugoslavian white and the sparkled arctic whiteness of Alexandrian white. Softening this expanse is a lovely oyster shade of velour carpeting — also seam-free as if a thick liquid velour squeegeed exactly evenly across the marble as the French would have squeegeed their crêpe batters across the rim-free surfaces of their crêpe irons. Returning to the carpet, there is a sense of magic and joy for my barefeet and it seems that I am dressed in chiffon-fluid Grecian garb, Isadora Duncan style. Especially, I'm remembering the transporting quality of the familiar strains of Mozart and Beethoven — first and second movements of piano concertos, it seems, perhaps Mozart's Twenty-First and Beethoven's Second and Third — and as I reflect on it, it seems that it is all fundamentally part of just what is and always is, so that I can't imagine before or beyond this sound-joy — as if present, past and future are linked inseparably. I notice in revisiting my **corridor** the curious absence of any sense of aroma, and I remember how unusual it had

---

[1] Transcribed meditation 9 July 2004 as part of Dr. Christine Page's seminar, *Navigating the Soul's Journey*, Level I Seminar, 8-11 July 2004. (Also please see *Sources Cited* under Page.)

[2] The **corridor** represents either where you are currently in your life or the past. The door is the initiation and the far side of the door represents one's future. Please consider that the corridor is as important as anything else and that the same applies both to the details of one's door and to the way in which one opens it. In short, the nuances both supplement and create one's mediation and the informations it is sharing.

also seemed at the time of the mediation. . . . Now I see myself walking towards the far wall in which we as a class have been told there is a door that we're to open and step through; however, I am not seeing a door in the expanse of white and with further concentration, I'm noticing that the expanse of white isn't a wall but rather a diaphanous manifestation of white — diaphanous though without being fabric or veil or curtain either. I have a sense of needing to move towards it anyway as we've been instructed to describe the terrain on the other side of this door I also can't see. Somehow I'm just trusting, knowing that even without the four-cornered definition of door-ness, something about that diaphanous expanse of white assures me that it is penetrable. And as I draw closer, indeed yes — it is of a density unlike mist or haze — denser somehow while retaining that quality of diaphanous without being fabric — a coloured translucence of that exquisite viscosity of the halo around lilaced pink neon and soft Ceylonese sapphire neon as the flow around the tubing becomes more etherically dense and cascades across the whiteness of a wall while still maintaining its ethereal palette — colours we don't usually know on Earth except in that ethereal inch or two extending beyond neon's tubing. It's about the quality of the light I guess — as if you could mix an ethereal creaminess[3] into the light much the way sherbet differs from sorbet and much the way the fruit-flavoured tropical lifesavers in cantaloupes and tangerine differ from the more transparent colours of the citrus ones in the five-flavoured rolls. Perhaps it would be something like maintaining the colour density of an intense rainbow when seen from a distance while adding just a hint of creaminess (again, creamy's density and not her colour) — but the palette would require touch-ups in the directions of peach and lime, aqua and lavender, silver, pink, and iridescence.
. . . Returning first, though, to those photo-real frames preceding these descriptive nuances of colour's texture — the diaphanous wall before me becomes (as so different from the wall across which colours play) — indeed becomes soft, fragile, white cream-dense aquas gently shifting through the barely pink of Howard Johnson peppermint without moving through or seeming to need to move through blues and violets — undulating fragiles of cantaloupe creams and melting dreamsicles shifting Escher-style into pinks as if they were the lateral perimeter of an Aalto vase. And as I step through the non-wall of light, it's like a fog-veil after all — the way moving into and through the earth-touching segment of a rainbow critically shifts from the touchable of colours seen from a distance to the gossamer particulate mists of interdimensional doorways and portals. And on the other side, everything bathes in liquid light — liquid lavenders, pinks, aquas, and emeralds hovering just barely on this side of lime. Wonderful children are hunched down to play with the fairies and the nymphs; indeed, it's like walking through a most wonderful fairytale of trees and roots and children playing with their fairy friends and elfin beings and there is such a remarkable fragrance at last — as if a noticeably missing dimension has been returned. All the white blossoms known for their fragrance are there — roses and hyacinths, freesias and jasmines, honeysuckles, magnolias, and lillies-of-the-valley. And it strikes me particularly that there doesn't seem to be any sense of

---

[3] Where creaminess references viscosity and a liquid's texture rather than her colour.

walls, just this fantasy — this fairytale world extending as far as I can see or sense and there is such an overwhelming experience of the forest floor being everywhere at the same level. It slippers across my mind that there is something here for the purpose of teaching me that the fairyworld co-exists with all other layers of perceivable realities and co-exists seamlessly and continuously whether we can always visually see this devic realm or not — much like the wondrous continuity and the *ever-* and *omni-*presence of synchronicity however punctuated, erratic, and discontinuous our conscious glimpses of her may be.

part the fourth:

———————

sources cited

celebrating guidance, abundance and life-altering thoughts

sources cited

books

Braden, Gregg. *Walking Between the Worlds: the Science of Compassion.* Bellevue, Washington: Radio Bookstore Press, 1997.

Buhner, Stephen Harrod. *The Lost Language of Plants: The Ecological Importance of Plant Medicines to Life on Earth.* White River Junction, Vermont: Chelsea Green Publishing Company, 2002.

Clark, Nancy Ann. *Earth in Ascension.* Tucson, Arizona: Violet Fire Publishing, 1995.

Cousens, Gabriel, M.D., M.D.(H), D.D. *Spiritual Nutrition and the Rainbow Diet.* San Rafael, California: Cassandra Press, 1986.

Crow, David. *In Search of the Medicine Buddha: A Himalayan Journey.* New York: Jeremy P. Tarcher/Putnam a member of Penguin Putnam, 2000.

Dewhurst-Maddock, Olivea. *The Book of Sound Therapy: Heal Yourself with Music and Voice.* New York City: Fireside, a division of Simon and Schuster, 1993.

Essene, Virginia, and Irving Feurst. *Energy Blessings from the Stars: Seven Initiations.* Santa Clara, California: Spiritual Education Endeavors Publishing Company, 1998.

Essene, Virginia, and Sheldon Nidle. *You are Becoming a Galactic Human.* Santa Clara, California: Spiritual Education Endeavors Publishing Company, 1994.

Lawlor, Robert. *Sacred Geometry: Philosophy and Practice.* New York City: Thames and Hudson Inc., 1982.

Lindlahr, Henry, M.D. *Philosophy of Natural Therapeutics.* Ed. and rev. Jocelyn C. D. Proby. Essex, England: C.W. Daniel Company Ltd., 2000.

Page, Dr. Christine. *Spiritual Alchemy: How to Transform Your Life.* Essex, England: C.W. Daniel Company Ltd., 2003.

Polich, Judith Bluestone. *Return of the Children of Light: Incan and Mayan Prophecies for a New World.* Rochester, Vermont: Bear and Company, 2001.

Wagner, David, and Gabriel Cousens, M.D. *Tachyon Energy: A New Paradigm in Holistic Healing.* Berkeley, California: North Atlantic Books, 1999.

With, Barbara. *Party of Twelve: The Afterlife Interviews.* La Pointe, Winsconsin: Mad Island Communications, 1999.

Wright, Machaelle Small. *Co-Creative Science: A Revolution in Science Providing Real Solutions for Today's Health and Environment.* Warrenton, Virginia: Perelandra, Ltd., 1997.

courses, discussions, and seminars

Biogenesis Advanced Training Seminar. (use of Atlanean energy programmed crystal tools and discs). Peaceful Meadow Retreat, Boulder, Colorado. 30 Aug. 2000.

Bryant, Susan. *Higher Realms of Dowsing Seminar.* Flagstaff, Arizona. 9 June 2001.

Crow, David. *In the Garden with the Medicine Buddha.* Introductory Evening Pre-seminar. Crestone Community Building, Crestone, Colorado. 28 June 2004.

- - - . *Pharmacy of Flowers Seminar.* Crestone Community Building, Crestone, Colorado. 29 June 2004.

Detzler, Robert E. *Spiritual Response Therapy Advanced Training Class.* Dallas, Texas. Sept. 2000.

- - - . *Spiritual Restructuring, Restructuring Healing Class.* Dallas, Texas. Oct. 2000.

Kapp, Barry, Master Medicinal Aromatherapist, and Audre Wenzler, Certified Medicinal Aromatherapist. *Medicinal Aromatherapy, Level I Seminar.* 2680 North Page Springs Road, Cornville, Arizona. 4-5 Jan. 2003.

- - - . *Advanced Medicinal Aromatherapy, Level II Seminar.* 2680 North Page Springs Road, Cornville, Arizona. 24-28 Mar. 2004.

Kroeger, Hanna, and teaching staff. *Natural and Spiritual Healing, Levels I and II Curriculum.* Peaceful Meadow Retreat, Boulder, Colorado. June 2000.

- - - . *Natural and Spiritual Healing, Level III Curriculum.* Peaceful Meadow Retreat, Boulder, Colorado. July 2000.

Page, Christine, M.D., Mystical Physician, Intuitive, and Homeopath. *Navigating the Soul's Journey, Level I Seminar.* The Hotel Santa Fe, Santa Fe, New Mexico. 8-11 July 2004.

Phillips, Charles Simon. Discussion with author referencing *The Continuum of Physics.* Crestone, Colorado. 21 Aug. 2004.

- - - . Discussion with author referencing *The Co-existence of Emotional Transference in Iatrogenic Settings.* Crestone, Colorado. 21 Aug. 2004.

Stevens, Robert, N.D., NTS(1-68), Director of NMSNT and Instructor. *Core Synchronism I.* New Mexico School of Natural Therapeutics, Albuquerque, New Mexico. 14-18 Aug. 2000.

- - - . *Core Synchronism II.* New Mexico School of Natural Therapeutics, Albuquerque, New Mexico. 21-25 Aug. 2000.

- - - . *Subtle Body Analysis (Radionics).* New Mexico School of Natural Therapeutics, Albuquerque, New Mexico. Sept. 2002.

- - - . *Reflexology and Reflex Polarity.* New Mexico School of Natural Therapeutics, Albuquerque, New Mexico. May. 2004.

- - - . *Nature Cure Applications.* New Mexico School of Natural Therapeutics, Albuquerque, New Mexico. 19 June 2004.

Taliaferro, The Rev. Albert Achilles, F.R.C., D.D. *Classes and study groups.* Homes of Jimmie Laurence, Kay Everett, and Betty Alexander, Dallas, Texas. 1961-1970 and 1972-1974.

Thayer, Stevan J. *Integrated Energy Therapy, Basic Level Curriculum.* Peaceful Meadow Retreat, Boulder, Colorado. June 2000.

- - - . *Integrated Energy Therapy, Intermediate Level Curriculum.* Peaceful Meadow Retreat, Boulder, Colorado. Aug. 2000.

- - - . *Integrated Energy Therapy, Advanced Level Curriculum.* Peaceful Meadow Retreat, Boulder, Colorado. Aug. 2000.

part the fifth:

other readings and visuals

a celebration of options

sketching again: visions of forward and the sacrament of choice

It is not easy for persons to make the time or even to choose to make the time, given their work and their family's schedules, to read or to inform themselves through direct or channeled meditations or through meditative time with texts read or discs seen or heard. Notwithstanding, there is today greater availability and greater ease of access to spiritual studies, channeled information, and guided meditations to help us unveil the realities of subtle energy and of ourselves as galactic beings. I am hopeful that the excerpts you have just read can serve as shortcuts and as possible tools for locating further readings, in case any of those included have evoked greater interest or an etheric connection of resonant response. Similarly, and by way of introduction to the following supplementary reading list, I am again as hopeful that the eclectic assemblage of titles next ahead can and will serve valuably and in tandem with the excerpts.

blessings and love . . .

supplementary readings and visuals

earth energies, sacred sites and geometries

Belle, Maureen L. *Gaiamancy: Creating Harmonious Environments*

Collinge, William. *Subtle Energy: Awakening to the Unseen Forces in Our Lives*

Cowan, David, and Rodney Girdlestone. *Safe As Houses?: Ill Health and Electro-stress in the Home*

Crisp, Roger. *Ley Lines of Wessex*

Devereux, Paul. *Haunted Land: Investigations into Ancient Mysteries and Modern Day Phenomena*

- - - . *The New Ley Hunter's Guide*

- - - . *Shamanism and the Mystery Lines: Ley Lines, Spirit Paths, Shape-Shifting and Out-of-Body Travel*

Leviton, Richard. *The Galaxy on Earth*

Little, Gregory L., prod. and nar. *Mound Builders: Edgar Cayce's Forgotten Legacy*. DVD

Little, Gregory L., John Van Auken, and Lora Little. *Mound Builders: Edgar Cayce's Forgotten Record of Ancient America*

Miller, Hamish, and Paul Broadhurst. *The Sun and the Serpent*

Munck, Carl. *The Code - Ancient Advanced Technology and the Global Earth Matrix.* 4 part series on DVD

Pennick, Nigel. *Sacred Geometry*

Street, C.E. *Earthstars: The Geometric Groundplan Underlying London's Ancient Sacred Sites and Its Significance for the New Age*

- - - . *Earthstars – The Visionary Landscape, Part One: London, City of Revelation*

Thurnell-Read, Jane. *Geopathic Stress: How Earth Energies Affect Our Lives*

William, Henry. *The American Rite.* DVD

- - - . *Secrets of the Bird Tribe.* DVD

- - - . *Stargate Mythology.* 6 pack DVD special:
  Anointing of the Dove
  Stairway to Heaven
  Starwalkers and the Dimensions of the Blessed
  Stargate 2012
  Lost Secrets of Jesus: The Wand and the Ring
  The Light Body Effect

the *new* energy

Begich, Nick, Ph.D. (Medicina Alternativa), and Jeane Manning. *Angels Don't Play this H.A.A.R.P.: Advances in Tesla Technology*

Braden, Gregg. *The Divine Matrix: Bridging Time, Space, Miracles, and Belief*

- - - . *The Language of the Divine Matrix.* DVD

- - - . *The Science of Miracles: The Quantum Language of Healing, Peace, Feeling, and Belief,* an illustrated interview with Braden. DVD

supplementary readings and visuals

Childress, David Hatcher. *Anti-Gravity and the World Grid: The Enlightened Environmental Theories of Viktor Schauberger*

- - - . *Anti-Gravity and the World Grid.* DVD

- - - . *The Free Energy Device Handbook*

Childress, David Hatcher, Christopher Dunn, Hal Fox, Doug Kenyon, et al. *Clash of the Geniuses: Inventing the Impossible.* DVD

Coats, Callum. *Sacred Living Geometry*

Free Energy: The Race to Zero Point. DVD

Holes in Heaven?. H.A.A.R.P. and Advances in Tesla Technology. Nar. by Martin Sheen. DVD

Lipton, Bruce H., Ph.D., William A. Tiller, Ph.D., and John Gray, Ph.D. *Quantum Communication.* Prod. David Sereda. DVD

Manning, Jeane. *The Coming Energy Revolution: The Search for Free Energy*

McTaggart, Lynne. *The Field: The Quest for the Secret Force of the Universe*

- - - . *The Intention Experiment: Using Your Thoughts to Change Your Life and the World*

McTaggart, Lynne, Bruce H. Lipton, Ph.D., and Eric Pearl, D.C. *The Living Matrix: The New Science of Healing.* DVD

Measuring the Immeasurable: The Scientific Case for Spirituality. Comp. Sounds True.

Miller, William R., Ph.D., and Janet C' de Baca, Ph.D. *Quantum Change: When Epiphanies and Sudden Insights Transform Ordinary Lives*

Nieper, Hans A. *Dr. Nieper's Revolution in Technology, Medicine and Society*

Radin, Dean, M.S. (Electrical Engineering), Ph.D. (Psychology). *The Conscious Universe: The Scientific Truth of Psychic Phenomena*

- - - . *Entangled Minds: Extrasensory Experiences in a Quantum Reality*

Schwartz, Gary E., Ph.D., and Linda Russek, Ph.D. *The Living Energy Universe: A Fundamental Discovery that Transforms Science and Medicine*

Wall, Ernst L., Ph.D. (Physics). *The Physics of Tachyons*

What the Bleep Do We Know!?. DVD

What the Bleep!? – Down the Rabbit Hole. DVD

Wilson, Edward O., Ph.D. (Biology), Entomologist and Sociobiologist. *Consilience: The Unity of Knowledge*

Zahourek, Rothlyn, R.N., Ph.D. *Intentionality: The Matrix of Healing: A Qualitative Theory for Research, Education and Practice*

Zohar, Danah. *The Quantum Self: Human Nature and Consciousness Defined by the New Physics*

Zohar, Danah, and Ian Marshall. *The Quantum Society: Mind, Physics, and a New Social Vision*

the Shift

Bourne, Edmund J., Ph.D. (Clinical Psychology). *Global Shift: How a New World View is Transforming Humanity*

Braden, Gregg. *Beyond Zero Point: The Journey of Compassion*. DVD

- - - . *Fractal Time: The Secret of 2012 and a New World Age*

Laszlo, Ervin, Ph.D. (Philosophy and Human Sciences), and 4 Hon. Ph.D.s. *Quantum Shift in the Global Brain*

Lipton, Bruce H., Ph.D., and Steve Bhaerman. *Spontaneous Evolution: Our Positive Future (and a Way to Get There from Here)*

Page, Christine, M.D., Mystical Physician, Intuitive, and Homeopath. *2012 and the Galactic Center: The Return of the Great Mother*

South, Stephanie. *2012: Biography of a Time Traveler: The Journey of José Argüelles*

Tart, Charles T., Ph.D. (Psychology). *The End of Materialism*

Vallée, Martine, ed. with Lee Carroll channeling Kryon, Tom Kenyon channeling the Hathors, and Patricia Cori channeling the High Council of Sirius. *The Great Shift: Co-Creating a New World for 2012 and Beyond*

Vallée, Martine, ed. with Lee Carroll channeling Kryon, Patricia Cori channeling the High Council of Sirius, and Pepper Lewis channeling Gaia. *Transition Now: Redefining Duality, 2012 and Beyond*

esoteric christianity

Baigent, Michael. *The Jesus Papers: Exposing the Greatest Cover-Up in History*

Baigent, Michael, Richard Leigh, and Henry Lincoln. *Holy Blood, Holy Grail*

Barnstone, Willis, and Marvin Meyer, eds. *The Gnostic Bible: Gnostic Texts of Mystical Wisdom from the Ancient and Medieval Worlds*

Besant, Annie. *Esoteric Christianity: The Lesser Mysteries*

Bunick, Nick. *In God's Truth*

Douglas-Klotz, Neil, Ph.D. (Religious Studies and Psychology). *Blessings of the Cosmos: Benedictions from the Aramaic Words of Jesus*

- - - . *The Hidden Gospel: Decoding the Spiritual Message of the Aramaic Jesus*

- - - . *Prayers of the Cosmos: Meditations on the Aramaic Words of Jesus*

Gardner, Lawrence. *Bloodline of the Holy Grail: the Hidden Lineage of Jesus Revealed*

- - - . *Genesis of the Grail Kings*

- - - . *The Magdalene Legacy*

Hammer, Marc. *The Jeshua Letters*

Heline, Corinne. *The Blessed Virgin Mary: Her Life and Mission*

- - - . *Mystic Masonry and the Bible*

- - - . The *New Age Bible Interpretations, Vols. 1-7 (especially Vols. 5 and 7)*
    Vol. 5: *The Chirst and His Mission*
    Vol. 7: *Mystery of the Christos*

- - - . *Questions and Answers on the Bible*

- - - . *The Bible and the Tarot*

Heline, Theodore. *Dead Sea Scrolls*

- - - . *Saint Francis, The Wolf of Gubbio*

Hodson, Geoffrey. *Hidden Wisdom in the Holy Bible, Vols. 1-4*

Hurtak, James J, Ph.D. (Social Science), Ph.D. (History). *The Pistis Sophia: A Coptic Gnostic Text with Commentary*

Kenyon, Tom, and Judy Sion. *The Magdalene Manuscript: Alchemies of Homer and the Sex Magic of Isis*

Lewis, H. Spencer. *The Mystical Life of Jesus*

Meyer, Marvin W., Ph.D. (Early Christian Studies). *The Gnostic Gospels of Jesus*

- - - . *The Gospels of Mary: The Secret Tradition of Mary Magdalene*

- - - , trans., intro., and notes. *The Secret Teachings of Jesus: Four Gnostic Gospels*

Newman, Sharon. *The Real History Behind the Da Vinci Code*

Pagels, Elaine, Ph.D. (Religious Studies). *Beyond Belief: The Secret Gospel of Thomas*

- - - . *The Gnostic Gospels*

- - - . *Gnostic Paul*

- - - . *Nag Hammadi Scriptures*

- - - . *The Origin of Satan*

- - - . *Reading Judas*

- - - . *Secrets of Mary Magdalene*

Picknett, Lynn. *Mary Magdalene*

Powell, Robert. *The Sophia Teachings: The Emergence of the Divine Feminine in Our Time*

- - - . *The Sophia Teachings: The Emergence of the Divine Feminine in Our Time.* 6 tape series

The Scrolls of Adam and Eve. Commentary by Dr. James J. Hurtak

Székely, Edmond Bordeaux, trans. and ed. *The Essene Gospel of Peace, Books 1-4:*
- 1. *Book One*
- 2. *The Unknown Books of the Essenes*
- 3. *Lost Scrolls of the Essene Brotherhood*
- 4. *The Teachings of the Elect*

Steiner, Rudolph, Ph.D. (Philosophy). *Isis Mary Sophia: Her Mission and Ours*

Taliaferro, A. A., F.R.C., D.D. *The Heart is the Manger: Sermons on the Incarnation*

- - - . *Sermons for Lent*

Valantasis, Richard. *Beliefnet Guide to Gnosticism and Other Vanished Christianities*

Wentworth, Adrienne. *Divine Intention: The Story of the Luciferian Conspiracy and God's Solutions*

reincarnation

Altea, Rosemary. *The Eagle and the Rose*

- - - . *A Matter of Life and Death: Remarkable True Stories of Hope and Healing*

Anderson, George, and Andrew Barone. *George Anderson's Lessons from the Light*

Anderson, Mary, Ph.D. *Awaken to Your Soul: A Guide to Remembering Who You Really Are*

Atwater, P.M.H. *The Big Book of Near Death Experiences*

Bache, Christopher M. *Life Cycles: Reincarnation and the Web of Life*

Beaconsfield, Hannah. *Welcome to Planet Earth: A Guide for Walk-Ins, Starseeds, and Lightworkers of all Varieties*

Bernard, Graham, channeled by. *Why You Are Who You Are: A Psychic Conversation*

supplementary readings and visuals

Borgia, Anthony. *Life in the World Unseen*

Browne, Sylvia. *Temples on the Other Side: How Wisdom from "Beyond the Veil" Can Help You Right Now*

Canon, Dolores. *Keepers of the Garden*

Caskey, Margaret. *The Third Choice: Walk-ins, Reincarnation, and a Spiritual Alternative to Human Suffering*

David, William, and Margaret Gibson. *Reincarnation and the Soul in the Parables of Jesus*

Katz, Ginny. *Beyond the Light*

MacGregor, Geddes, D.D., D. Phil. (Oxon). *Reincarnation in Christianity*

McKnight, Rosalind A. *Soul Journeys: My Guided Tours through the Afterlife*

Moody, Raymond A., Jr., M.D., Ph.D., with Brian L. Weiss, M.D. *Life Between Life*

Newton, Michael, Ph.D. (Counseling Psychology), Cert. Master Hyp. *Destiny of Souls*

- - - . *Journey of Souls*

Roberts, Jane. *The Oversoul Seven Trilogy:*
   1. *The Education of Oversoul Seven*
   2. *The Further Education of Oversoul Seven*
   3. *Oversoul Seven and the Museum of Time*

Ward, Suzanne. *Matthew, Tell Me about Heaven*

Ward, Sylvia, with Avril Newey. *The Clew*

Weiss, Brian L., M.D. *Many Lives, Many Masters*

- - - . *Messages from the Masters: Tapping into the Power of Love*

unfolding the cosmic tapestry

Archangel Ariel channeled by Tachi-Ren. *What is Lightbody?*

Ardagh, Arjuna. *Awakening Into Oneness: The Power of Blessing in the Evolution of Consciousness*

Bailey, Alice A., received and edited by. *Esoteric Astrology*

- - - , received and edited by. *Esoteric Psychology*

- - - , received and edited by. *Letters on Occult Meditation*

- - - , received and edited by. *A Treatise on White Magic: The Way of the Disciple*

Bailey, Alice A. *Ponder This: A Compilation from the Writings of Alice Bailey and the Tibetan Master Djwhal Khul.* Comp. by a student

Baumann, T. Lee, M.D. *God at the Speed of Light: The Melding of Science and Spirituality*

Berges, John. *Sacred Vessel of the Mysteries: The Great Invocation, Word of Power, Gift of Love*

Braden, Gregg. *Awakening to Zero Point: The Collective Initiative*

- - - . *The God Code: The Secret of Our Past, the Promise of Our Future*

- - - . *The Isaiah Effect: Decoding the Lost Science of Prayer and Prophecy*

- - - . *Lost Mode of Prayer.* Audio book on CD

- - - . *Secrets of the Lost Mode of Prayer: The Hidden Power of Beauty, Blessings, Wisdom, and Hurt*

- - - . *Walking Between the Worlds: The Science of Compassion*

- - - . *Walking Between the Worlds: Understanidng the Inner Technology of Emotion.* 2 DVD set

supplementary readings and visuals

Bryce, Sheradon, channeled by. *Joy Riding the Universe: Snapshots of the Journey, Vol. I*

Byrne, Rhonda. *The Secret*

Carey, Ken. *The Third Millennium: Living in the Posthistoric World*

Clark, Glenn. *The Man Who Tapped the Secrets of the Universe*

Clow, Barbara Hand. *Catastrophobia: The Truth Behind Earth Changes in the Coming Age of Light*

Cox, Robert. *The Pillar of Celestial Fire: The Lost Science of the Ancient Seers Rediscovered*

De Mello, Anthony. *Awareness: The Perils and Opportunities of Reality*

Detzler, Robert E. *Soul Re-Creation: Developing Your Cosmic Potential*

Doreal, Dr. M., trans. and interp. *The Emerald Tablets of Thoth, the Atlantean*

Elliott, William. *Tying Rocks to Clouds: Meetings and Conversations with Wise and Spiritual People*

Emoto, Masaru, Doctor of Alternative Medicine. *The Hidden Messages in Water*

- - - . *The Hidden Messages in Water*. DVD

- - - . *Messages from Water*. DVD

Essene, Virginia. *Secret Truths: A Young Adult's Guide for Creating Peace*

Gire, Ken. *Seeing What is Sacred: Becoming More Spiritually Sensitive to Everyday Moments of Life*

- - - . *Windows of the Soul: Experiencing God in New Ways*

Grof, Stanislav, M.D., Ph.D. (Medicine). *The Consciousness Revolution: A Transatlantic Dialogue* (two days with Stanislav Grof, Ervin Laszlo, and Peter Russell)

- - - . *The Transpersonal Vision: The Healing Potential of Non-Ordinary States of Consciousness*

- - - . *When the Impossible Happens: Adventures in Non-Ordinary Reality*

Grof, Stanislav, M.D., Ph.D., with Hal Zina Bennett. *The Holotropic Mind: The Three Levels of Consciousness and How They Shape Our Lives*

Hawkins, David R., M.D., Ph.D. *Transcending Levels of Consciousness*

Heline, Corinne. *America's Invisible Guidance*

Heline, Theodore. *Archetypes Unveiled*

Hilarion, transmitted through Maurice B. Cooke. *Astrology Plus*

- - - , transmitted through Maurice B. Cooke. *The Nature of Reality: A Book of Explanations*

- - - , transmitted through Maurice B. Cooke. *Seasons of the Spirit*

- - - , transmitted through Maurice B. Cooke. *Symbols*

- - - , transmitted through Maurice B. Cooke. *Threshold: A Letter for Michelle, from Hilarion*

Hodson, Geoffrey. *Clairvoyant Investigations*

Hurtak, James J, Ph.D. (Social Science), Ph.D. (History). *The Book of Knowledge: The Keys of Enoch*

Karpinski, Gloria. *Barefoot on Holy Ground*

- - - . *Where Two Worlds Touch*

King, Godfrey Ray. *The Magic Presence*, No.2 in St. Germain Series

- - - . *Unveiled Mysteries*, No.1 in St. Germain Series

supplementary readings and visuals

Krippner, Stanley, Ph.D. (Psychology), and Harris L. Friedman, Ph.D. (Educational Psychology), eds. *Mysterious Minds: The Neurobiology of Psychics, Mediums and Other Extraordinary People*

LaBerge, Stephen, Ph.D. (Psychophysiology). *Lucid Dreaming: A Concise Guide to Awakening in Your Dreams and in Your Life*

LaBerge, Stephen, Ph.D., and Howard Rheingold. *Exploring the World of Lucid Dreaming*

Laszlo, Ervin, Ph.D. (Philosophy and Human Sciences), and 4 Hon. Ph.D.s. *Science and the Akashic Field: An Integral Theory of Everything*

Leadbeater, Charles W. *The Inner Life*

Lumari. *Akashic Records: Collective Keeper of Divine Expression*

Martin, Lin David. *Divine Chuckles: Life from a Higher Perspective*

Milanovich, Norma J., Ph.D., and Shirley D. McCune, Ph.D. *The Light Shall Set You Free*

Miller, Patrick D. *The Complete Story of the Course: The History, the People, and the Controversies Behind A Course in Miracles*

Millman, Dan. *Living on Purpose: Straight Answers to Life's Tough Questions*

Northrop, Suzane. *Everything Happens for a Reason*

Pearce, Joseph Chilton. *The Biology of Transcendence: A Blueprint of the Human Spirit*

Petrovic, John Joseph, Ph.D. *The First Principles: A Scientist's Guide to the Spiritual*

Pons, Dale, Edgar Cayce, John Keely, Rudolf Steiner, and Nikola Tesla. *The Physics of Love: the Ultimate Universal Laws*

Rasha, received and transcribed by. *Oneness: The Teachings*

Robinson, Suzanne. *Soul Gardening: The Sacred Art of Relating Harmoniously*

Rudhyar, Dane. *The Planetarization of Consciousness*

Russell, Walter. *The Secret of Life*

Ryder, Ruth, channeled by, from information received from the higher dimensional master teachers Peter, Sawanda, Hilarion, Katherine, William, and Marian. *The Golden Path: An Introduction to Advanced Spiritual Knowledge*

Schlemmer, Phyllis V., and Palden Jenkins. *The Only Planet of Choice: Essential Briefings from Deep Space*

Schlitz, Marilyn Mandala, Ph.D., Casandra Vieten, Ph.D., and Tina Amorok, Psy.D. *Living Deeply: The Art and Science of Transformation in Everyday Life,* based on a 10 year research program at the Institute of Noetic Sciences

- - - . *Living Deeply: Transformative Practices From the World's Wisdom Traditions.* DVD

Senner, Madis. *The Way Home: Making Heaven on Earth*

Sheldrake, Rupert, Ph.D. (Biochemistry). *Seven Experiments That Could Change the World: A Do-It-Yourself Guide to Revolutionary Science*

Singer, Michael A. *The Untethered Soul: The Journey Beyond Yourself*

Solara. *The Star-Borne: A Remembrance for the Awakened Ones*

Steiner, Rudolf, Ph.D. (Philosophy). *Cosmic Memory: Atlantis and Lemuria*

Temple-Thurston, Leslie, with Brad Laughlin. *Returning to Oneness: The Seven Keys of Ascension*

Thayer, Stevan J., and Linda Sue Nathanson, Ph.D. *Interview with an Angel: Our World, Ourselves, Our Destiny,* as received from the Archangel Ariel

supplementary readings and visuals

Todeschi, Kevin J. *Edgar Cayce on the Akashic Records*

Tolle, Eckhart. *A New Earth: Awakening to Your Life's Purpose*

Twyman, James F. *The Moses Code*

- - - . *The Moses Code.* DVD

Virtue, Doreen, Ph.D. (Counseling Psychology). *The Lightworker's Way: Awakening Your Spiritual Power to Know and Heal*

Vywamus, channeled through Janet McClure. *Light Techniques that Trigger Transformation*

Ward, Suzanne. *Illuminations for a New Era*

- - - . *Revelations for a New Era*

- - - . *Voices of the Universe*

Wyllie, Timothy. *Dolphins, ETs, and Angels: Adventures Among Spiritual Intelligences*

Zukav, Gary. *The Secret of the Soul*

children

Atwater, P.M.H. *Beyond the Indigo Children: The New Children and the Coming of the Fifth World*

- - - . *Children of the New Millennium: Children's Near-Death Experiences and the Evolution of Humankind*

Bowan, Carol. *Children's Past Lives*

Katie, Byron, and Hans Wilhelm. *Tiger-Tiger, Is It True?: Four Questions to Make You Smile Again*

Hardo, Trutz. *Children Who Have Lived Before*

Martin, Joel, and Patricia Romanowski. *Our Children Forever: George Anderson's Messages from Children on the Other Side*

Peterson, James W. *The Secret Life of Kids: An Exploration Into Their Psychic Senses*

Sulara, Teran W. *Keys for Creating Your Life 1-4*

Tolle, Eckhart. *Milton's Secret*

Twyman James F. *Emissary of Love: The Psychic Children Speak to the World*

- - - . *Messages from Thomas: Raising Psychic Children*

Virtue, Doreen, Ph.D. (Counseling Psychology). *The Care and Feeding of Indigo Children*

- - - . *The Crystal Children: A Guide to the Newest Generation of Psychic and Sensitive Children*

intuition

Anderson, Ted. *More Simplified Magic: Pathworking and the Tree of Life*

Ashcroft-Nowicki, Delores. *Highways of the Mind: The Art and History of Pathworking*

Eyre, Richard. *Spiritual Serendipity: Cultivating and Celebrating the Art of the Unexpected*

Halberstam, Yitta, and Judith Leventhal. *Small Miracles: Extraordinary Coincidences from Everyday Life*

- - - . *Small Miracles II*

Keen, Linda. *Intuition Magic: Understanding Your Psychic Nature*

Naparstek, Belleruth. *Your Sixth Sense: Unlocking the Power of Your Intuition*

Orloff, Judith, M.D., Psychiatrist and Medical Intuitive. *Second Sight*

Page, Christine, M.D., Mystical Physician, Intuitive, and Homeopath. *Beyond the Obvious: Bringing Intuition into Our Awakening Consciousness*

Peat, F. David. *Synchronicity: The Bridge Between Matter and Mind*

Pierce, Penny. *The Intuitive Way: A Guide to Living from Inner Wisdom*

Thurston, Mark, D.C. *Synchronicity As Spiritual Guidance*

inspiration

Brewer, Anne. *Breaking Free to Health, Wealth and Happiness: 100's of Powerful Ways to Release Limiting Beliefs*

Carlson, Richard. *Don't Sweat the Small Stuff . . . and It's All Small Stuff*

Cates, David. *Unconditional Money: A Magical Journey Into the Heart of Abundance*

Cohen, Alan. *The Peace That You Seek*

Gaines, The Rev. Edwene. *The Four Spiritual Laws of Prosperity*

- - - . *Prosperity Affirmation Cards*

Mandino, Og. *The Greatest Miracle in the World*

Messages from the Universe. Oracle cards. © Les Éditions Universelles du Verseau

Millman, Dan, and Doug Childers. *Divine Interventions: True Stories of Mystery and Miracles that Change Lives*

Nerburn, Kent. *Small Graces: the Quiet Gifts of Everyday Life*

Price, John Randolph. *The Abundance Book*

Ruiz, Miguel. *The Four Agreements*

Yatek, Verna V., Kevin Ryerson, et al., trance channeled through these beings. *The Butterfly Rises: One Woman's Transformation Through the Trance Channeling of . . .*

angels and guides

Belhayes, Iris, and Enid. *Spirit Guides*

Fox, Matthew, Ph.D. (Spirituality), American Anglican Priest and Theologian, and Rupert Sheldrake, Ph.D. (Biochemistry). *The Physics of Angels*

Guillory, William A., Ph.D. (Physical Chemistry). *The Guides: Cameron, Lea, Aeschyleus*

Leadbeater, Charles W. *Invisible Helpers*

Petrak, Joyce, Doctor of Clinical Hypnotherapy. *Angels, Guides and Other Spirits: Incredible Events from the Unseen World Around Us as Told by a Spirit Release Therapist*

Virtue, Doreen, Ph.D. (Counseling Psychology). *Angels 101*

- - - . *Archangels and Ascended Masters*

- - - . *Healing with the Angels*

- - - . *Healing with the Angels.* Oracle cards

- - - . *Saints and Angels.* Oracle cards

Virtue, Doreen, Ph.D. (Counseling Psychology), with Amy Oscar. *My Guardian Angel*

Virtue, Doreen, Ph.D. (Counseling Psychology), and Charles Virtue, Angel Therapy Practitioner®. *Signs From Above*

Price, John Randolph. *The Angels Within Us*

Webster, Richard. *Spirit Guides and Angel Guardians*

White, Ruth. *Working with Your Guides and Angels*

Wülfing, Sulamith. *Angel Oracle*. Oracle cards. © Bluestar Communications Corp., 1997

Young, Meredith L., and Judi A. Winall. *Angelic Messenger Cards*

shamanism

Anderson, Lynn V. *The Woman of Wyrrd: The Arousal of the Inner Fire*

Andrews, Ted. *Animal Speak: The Spiritual and Magical Powers of Creatures Great and Small*

- - - . *Animal Wise: The Spirit Language and Signs of Nature*

Arrien, Angeles, Ph.D., and 4 Hon. Ph.D.s, Cultural Anthropologist. *The Four-Fold Way: Walking the Paths of the Warrior, Teacher, Healer, and Visionary*

Arvigo, Rosita, and Nadine Epstein. *Sastun: My Apprenticeship with a Maya Healer*

Capra, Fritjof, Ph.D., Physicist and Systems Theorist. *The Tao of Physics*

Carson, David, Jamie Sams, and Angela C. Werneke. *Medicine Cards: The Discovery of Power Through the Ways of Animals*

- - - . *Medicine Cards: The Discovery of Power Through the Ways of Animals*. the Cards

Conway, D.J. *Animal Magick*

Cowan, Eliot, Shaman (Huichol). *Plant Spirit Medicine: Healing with the Power of Plants*

Dolfyn. *Bough Down: Praying with Tree Spirits*

- - - . *Shamanism: A Beginners Guide*

- - - . *Shamanism and Nature Spirituality: The Sacred Circle*

- - - . *Shamanic Wisdom: Nature Spirituality, Sacred Power and Earth Ecstasy*

Espinoza, Luis (Chamalú). *Chamalú: The Shamanic Way of the Heart*

Gregg, Susan, Ph.D. (Clinical Hypnotherapy). *Dance of Power: A Shamanic Journey*

Harner, Michael, Ph.D. (Anthropology), Hon. Ph.D. (Shamanic Studies). *The Way of the Shaman*

Krippner, Stanley. Ph.D. (Educational Psychology). *Ayahuasca and Mystical Secrets of the Amazon*

Larsen, Stephen. *The Shaman's Doorway: Opening Imagination to Power and Myth*

Lorler, Marie-Lu. *Shamanic Healing Within the Medicine Wheel*

Perkins, John. *Psychonavigation: Techniques for Travel Beyond Time*

- - - . *The World is as You Dream It: Shamanic Teachings from the Amazon and Andes*

Schultes, Richard Evans, and Albert Hoffman, Ph.D. (Chemistry). *Plants of the Gods: Their Sacred, Healing, and Hallucinogenic Powers*

Stevens, José, and Lena Sedletzky Stevens. *Secrets of Shamanism: Tapping the Spirit Power Within You*

Sun Bear, and Waban. *The Medicine Wheel: Earth Astrology*

Villoldo, Alberto, Ph.D. (Psychology), and Erik Jendresen. *Dance of the Four Winds: Secrets of the Inca Medicine Wheel*

Villoldo, Alberto, Ph.D. (Psychology), and Stanley Krippner, Ph.D. (Educational Psychology). *Healing States: A Journey into the World of Spiritual Healing and Shamanism*

Weiss, Brian L., M.D. *Through Time into Healing*

Windwalker, Kiara. *Doorway to Consciousness*

entheogens

Jansen, Karl, M.D. *Ketamine: Dreams and Realities*

Ott, Jonathan. *The Age of Entheogens and the Angels' Dictionary*

- - - . *Pharmacophilia or the Natural Paradises*

Pendell, Dale. *Pharmako/Poeia: Plant Powers, Poisons, and Herbcraft*

Shulgin, Alexander, Ph.D. (Biochemistry). *Pihkal*

- - - . *Tihkal*

Weil, Andrew, M.D., and Winifred Rosen. *From Chocolate to Morphine: Everything You Need to Know about Mind-Altering Drugs*

animals

Bell, Kristen Leigh, Certified Master Aromatherapist. *Holistic Aromatherapy for Animals*

Boone, J. Allen. *Kinship with All Life*

Brady, Linda M., Marty Humphreys, and J. C. Landis. *No More Goodbyes*

Devi, Lila. *Flower Essences for Animals: Remedies for Helping the Pets You Love*

The Dolphin's Gift: How a Dolphin's Love Transformed the People of Dingle Bay. Nar. John Hurt. DVD

Graham, Helen, and Gregory Vlamis. *Bach Flower Remedies for Animals*

Kowalski, Gary. *The Souls of Animals*

Shapiro, Robert, and Julie Rapkin. *Awakening to the Animal Kingdom*

Sichel, Elaine, ed. *Circles of Compassion*

Smith, Penelope. *Animals . . . Our Return to Wholeness*

Summers, Patty. *Talking with Animals*

Thomas, Agnes J., Ph.D. *Pets Tell the Truth*

nature

Altman, Nathaniel. *The Deva Handbook: How to Work with Nature's Subtle Energies*

Callahan, Philip S., Ph.D. (Entomology). *Ancient Mysteries, Modern Visions: The Magnetic Life of Agriculture*

- - - . *Exploring the Spectrum*

- - - . *Tuning in to Nature: Infrared Radiation And the Insect Communication System*

The Findhorn Community. *The Findhorn Garden*

Heline, Corinne. *Magic Gardens*

- - - . *Star Gates*

Hodson, Geoffrey. *Fairies at Work and at Play*

- - - . *The Kingdom of the Gods*

Kelly, Penny. *The Elves of Lilly Hill Farm: A Partnership with Nature*

Kunz, Dora van Gelder. *Devic Consciousness*

- - - . *The Real World of Fairies: A First Person Account*

Leadbeater, Charles W. *The Hidden Side of Things*

Poganik, Marko. *Nature Spirits and Elemental Beings: Working with the Intelligence in Nature*

The Queen of Trees. Filmed, dir., writ. and prod. Mark Deeble and Victoria Stone. DVD

Shapiro, Robert, and Julie Rapkin. *Awakening to the Plant Kingdom*

Sheldrake, Rupert, Ph.D. (Biochemistry). *The Presence of the Past: Morphic Resonance and the Habits of Nature*

- - - . *The Rebirth of Nature: the Greening of Science and God*

Tompkins, Peter, and Christopher Bird. *The Secret Life of Plants*

Virtue, Doreen, Ph.D. (Counseling Psychology). *Fairies 101*

- - - . *Healing with the Fairies*

Wright, Machaelle Small. *Behaving As If the God in All Life Mattered*

wicca

Cunningham, Scott. *The Truth About Witchcraft Today*

- - - . *Wicca: A Guide for the Solitary Practitioner*

Curott, Phyllis. *Book of Shadows: A Modern Woman's Journey into the Wisdom of Witchcraft and the Magic of the Goddess*

Raven, Grimassi. *The Wiccan Mysteries: Ancient Origins and Teachings*

psychological health

Amen, Daniel G., M.D. *Change Your Brain, Change Your Body*

- - - . *Change Your Brain, Change Your Life*

Arbinger Institute. *The Anatomy of Peace: Resolving the Heart of Conflict*

Borysenko, Joan, Ph.D. (Medical Sciences). *Inner Peace for Busy People*

Braden, Gregg. *The Spontaneous Healing of Belief: Shattering the Paradigm of False Limits*

Carlson, Richard. *You Can be Happy No Matter What*

Cherry, David, and Marlene Miller. *Brain Styles*

Covey, Stephen R. *The 7 Habits of Highly Effective People: Powerful Lessons in Personal Change*

- - - . *The 8th Habit: From Effectiveness to Greatness*

Clynes, Manfred. *Sentics: The Touch of the Emotions*

Cytowic, Richard E., M.D., Neurologist. *The Man Who Tasted Shapes*

Day, Laura. *The Circle: How the Power of a Single Wish Can Change Your Life*

- - - . *Welcome to Your Crisis: How to Use the Power of Crisis to Create the Life You Want*

de Bergerac, Olivia. *The Dolphin Within*

supplementary readings and visuals

de Bono, Edward., Ph.D., D. Phil. (Medicine), D. Design, M.D. *Children Solve Problems*

- - - . *The Dog Exercising Machine*

- - - . *Lateral Thinking*

- - - . *Letters to Thinkers*

- - - . *PO: Beyond Yes and No*

Dispenza, Joe, D.C. *Evolve Your Brain: The Science of Changing Your Mind*

- - - . *Evolve Your Brain: The Science of Changing Your Mind.* DVD

Dossey, Larry, M.D. *Be Careful What You Pray For . . . You Just Might Get It*

- - - . *Healing Words: The Power of Prayer and the Practice of Medicine*

- - - . *Prayer is Good Medicine: How to Reap the Healing Benefits of Prayer*

Dwoskin, Hale. *The Sedona Method: Your Key to Lasting Happiness, Success, Peace, and Emotional Well-being*

Dyer, Wayne W., Ph.D. (Educational Counseling). *Change Your Thoughts, Change Your Life*

- - - . *Inspiration: Your Ultimate Calling*

- - - . *Power of Intention: Learning to Co-create Your World Your Way*

- - - . *Pulling Your Own Strings: Dynamic Techniques for Dealing with Other People and Living Your Life as You Choose*

- - - . *Real Magic: Creating Miracles in Everyday Life*

- - - . *There's a Spiritual Solution to Every Problem*

- - - . *There's a Spiritual Solution to Every Problem.* DVD

- - - . *You'll See It When You Believe It: The Way to Your Personal Transformation*

Fitzgerald, Michele K. *Chasing the Shadow of Free Will: An Introduction to Belief Codes*

Ford, Debbie. *The Right Questions*

Gibran, Kalil. *The Prophet*

Glaser, Aura., Ph.D. (Clinical Psychology). *A Call to Compassion: Bringing Buddhist Practices of the Heart into the Soul of Psychology*

Grabhorn, Lynn. *Excuse Me, Your Life is Waiting: The Astonishing Power of Feelings*

Grof, Stanislav, M.D., Ph.D. (Medicine), Psychiatrist. *Psychology of the Future: Lessons from Modern Consciousness Research*

Grof, Stanislav, M.D., Ph.D. (Medicine), Psychiatrist, with Christina Grof, Psychotherapist, eds. *Spiritual Emergency: When Personal Transformation Becomes a Crisis*

Hanh, Thich Nhat, Zen Master. *Being Peace*

Hawkins, David R., M.D., Ph.D. *I: Reality and Subjectivity*

- - - . *Power vs. Force: The Hidden Determinants of Human Behavior*

Hay, Louise L. *You Can Heal You Life*

Hay, Louise L., with Linda Carwin Tomchin. *The Power is Within You*

Hayward, Jeremy, with Karen Hayward. *Sacred World: A Guide to Shambhala Warriorship in Daily Life*

Hicks, Esther, and Jerry Hicks. *The Amazing Power of Deliberate Intent: Living the Art of Allowing*

- - - . *Ask And It Is Given: Learning to Manifest Your Desires*

- - - . *Ask And It Is Given.* the Cards

- - - . *The Astonishing Power of Emotions: Let Your Feelings Be Your Guide*

- - - . *The Law of Attraction: The Basics of the Teachings of Abraham*

- - - . *Let It Loose!: The Law of Attraction in Action — Episode X.* DVD

- - - . *The Vortex: Where the Law of Attraction Assembles All Cooperative Realationships*

- - - . *Who You Really Are!: The Law of Attraction in Action — Episode XI.* DVD

Jawer, Michael A., with Marc S. Micozzi, M.D., Ph.D. *The Spiritual Anatomy of Emotion: How Feelings Link the Brain, the Body, and the Sixth Sense*

Johnson, Debbie. *Think Yourself Loved*

Joy, W. Brugh, M.D. *Joy's Way*

Katie, Byron. *Who Would You Be Without Your Story?: Dialogues with Byron Katie*

Katie, Byron, with Michael Katz. *I Need Your Love — Is That True?: How to Stop Seeking Love, Approval, and Appreciation and Start Finding Them Instead*

Katie, Byron, and Stephen Mitchell. *Loving What Is: Four Questions That Can Change Your Life*

- - - . *A Thousand Names for Joy: Living in Harmony with the Way Things Are*

Kenyon, Tom. *Brain States*

Kirby, Maureen, Ph.D. *Why Are We Still Fighting?*

Kornfield, Jack. *The Wise Heart: A Guide to the Universal Teachings of Buddhist Psychology*

Laskow, Leonard, M.D. *Healing with Love: A Breakthrough Mind/Body Program for Healing Yourself and Others*

Lerner, Isha, and Mark Lerner. *Inner Child Cards: A Fairy-Tale Tarot*

- - - . *Inner Child Cards: A Fairy-Tale Tarot. the Cards.* Illus. Christopher Guilfoil

Lipton, Bruce H., Ph.D. (Cellular Biology). *The Biology of Belief: Unleashing the Power of Consciousness, Matter, and Miracles*

- - - . "Mind Over Genes: The New Biology." *Alternatives*. Winter 03-04, Issue 28. www.brucelipton.com.

- - - . *The Answer to Nature vs. Nurture.* CD

- - - . *Biology of Perception, The Psychology of Change.* CD

- - - . *Cellular Biology and Positive Thoughts.* CD

- - - . *The Science of Health.* CD

- - - . *Your Lifestyle Impacts Your Genetics.* CD

- - - . *Biology of Belief.* 4 DVDS
    1. *The New Biology*
    2. *The Biology of Perception, The Psychology of Change*
    3. *Nature, Nurture, and the Power of Love: Conscious Parenting*
    4. *As Above — So Below*

Millman, Dan. *No Ordinary Moments: A Peaceful Warrior's Guide to Daily Life*

Morrissey, Mary Manin. *Building Your Field of Dreams*

Murphy, Joseph. *The Power of Your Subconscious Mind*

- - - . *These Truths Can Change Your Life*

Murray, Pamela. *The New Success: How to Redefine, Create, and Survive Your Own Success*

Myss, Caroline. *Why People Don't Heal and How They Can*

Page, Christine, M.D., Mystical Physician, Intuitive, and Homeopath. *Frontiers of Health: From Healing to Wholeness*

- - - . *The Mirror of Existence: Stepping Into Wholeness*

Pearsall, Paul, Ph.D. (Neuropsychology). *The Beethoven Factor: The New Positive Psychology of Hardiness, Happiness, Healing and Hope*

- - - . *The Heart's Code: Tapping the Wisdom and Power of Our Heart Energy*

- - - . *Toxic Success: How to Stop Striving and Start Thriving*

Pert, Candace B., Ph.D. (Pharmacology), Neuropharmacologist. *Everything You Need to Know to Feel Go(o)d*

- - - . *The Molecules of Emotion*

Prem Raja Baba. *The Joy Book*

Richardson, Cheryl. *The Art of Extreme Self-Care*

- - - . *Create an Abundant Life*. DVD

- - - . *Life Makeovers*

- - - . *Stand Up for Your Life*

- - - . *Take Time for Your Life*

- - - . *The Unthinkable Touch of Grace: How to Recognize and Respond to the Spiritual Signposts in Your Life*

Rosenberg, Marshall B., Ph.D. (Clinical Psychology). *Non-Violent Communication: A Language of Life*

Sacks, Oliver, M.D., Neurologist. *The Man Who Mistook His Wife for a Hat: And Other Clinical Tales*

Schucman, Helen. *A Course in Miracles*

Seagram, Paol. *Socks in the Dryer*

Thurston, Mark, D.C., and Sarah Thurston. *Twelve Positive Habits of Spiritually Centered People: Simple Methods to Transform Your Life!*

Tipping, Colin C. *Radical Forgiveness: Making Room for the Miracle*

Truman, Karol K. *Feelings Buried Alive Never Die*

Zemke, The Rev. LeRoy E. *Thoughts for Transformation: Spiritual Insights for Positive Living*

Zukav, Gary and Linda Francis. *The Mind of the Soul*

health

Bailey, Alice, received and edited by. *Esoteric Healing*

Challoner, H.K. *The Path of Healing*

Chopra, Deepak, M.D. *Ageless Body, Timeless Mind: The Quantum Alternative to Growing Old*

- - - . *Creative Health: How to Wake Up the Body's Intelligence*

- - - . *Perfect Health: The Complete Mind/Body Guide*

- - - . *Quantum Healing: Exploring the Frontiers of Mind/Body Medicine*

supplementary readings and visuals

Cunningham, Donna, and Andrew Ramer. *Further Dimensions of Healing Addictions*

- - - . *The Spiritual Dimensions of Healing Addictions*

D'Adamo, Peter J., N.D. with Catherine Whitney. *4 Blood Types, 4 Diets: Eat Right for Your Type*

Cousens, Gabriel, M.D., M.D.(H), D.D. *Spiritual Nutrition and the Rainbow Diet*

Essene, Virginia, ed. *New Cells, New Bodies, New Life!: You're Becoming a Fountain of Youth!*

Fuhrman, Joel., M.D. *Eat to Live*

Heline, Corinne. *Occult Anatomy and the Bible*

Horowitz, Leonard G., D.M.D., M.P.H. *In Lies We Trust:* Documentary

Horowitz, Leonard G., D.M.D., M.P.H., and Joseph E. Barber, Ph.D. (Psychology). *The Healing Codes for the Biological Apocalypse*

Huddleston, Peggy. *Prepare for Surgery, Heal Faster: A Guide of Mind-Body Techniques*

Karagulla, Shafica, M.D., and Dora van Gelder Kunz. *The Chakras and the Human Energy Fields*

Kliment, Felicia Drury. *The Acid-Alkaline Balance Diet*

Kroeger, The Rev. Hanna. *The Seven Spiritual Causes of Ill Health*

Lappé, Marc, Ph.D., Educator, Toxicologist and Medical Ethicist. *When Antibiotics Fail: Restoring the Ecology of the Body*

Miller, Neil Z. *Immunization Theory vs. Reality*

- - - . *Vaccines: Are They Really Safe and Effective?*

Oyle, Irving, M.D. *The Healing Mind*

- - - . *Magic, Mysticism, and Modern Medicine: Journal of a Family Physician*

- - - . *The New American Medicine Show*

- - - . *Time, Space and the Mind*

- - - . *The Wizdom Within: On Daydreams, Realities, and Revelations*

Page, Christine, M.D., and Keith Hagenbach. *Mind, Body, Spirit Workbook: A Handbook for Health*

Pert, Candace B., Ph.D. (Pharmacology), Neuropharmacologist. *Your Body Is Your Subconscious Mind.* 3 CDs

Schlitz, Marilyn Mandala, Ph.D., and Tina Amorok, Psy.D. with Marc S. Micozzi, M.D., Ph.D. *Consciousness and Healing: Integral Approaches to Mind-Body Medicine*

Shealy, Norman C., M.D. *Sacred Healing, the Curing Power of Energy and Spirituality*

Stewart, William B., M.D. *Deep Medicine: Harnessing the Source of Your Healing Power*

Yiamonyiannis, John, Ph.D. (Biochemistry). *Fluoride the Aging Factor: How to Recognize and Avoid the Devastating Effects of Fluoride*

healers

Adam. *DreamHealer: His Name is Adam*

- - - . *DreamHealer 2: Guide to Self Empowerment*

Calvert, Peter. *Guided Healing: The Art of Transferring Love Between Realms*

supplementary readings and visuals

Diamond, John, M.D., Dip. (Psychological Medicine), Holistic Psychiatrist and Physician. *Facets of a Diamond: Reflections of a Healer*

Dr. Fritz - Healing the Body and Spirit. Documentary by David Sonnenschein. Videocassette

Hamilton, Allan J., M.D. *The Scalpel and the Soul: Encounters with Surgery, the Supernatural, and the Healing Power of Hope*

Henry, Ronald, with Kevin Ryerson. *The Future Healer: Spirit Communication on Healing*

Holzer, Hans. *The Secret of Healing: The Healing Powers of Ze'ev Kolman*

Maki, Masao. *In Search of Brazil's Quantum Surgeon: The Dr. Fritz Phenomenon*

Nani, Christel. *Diary of a Medical Intuitive*

Willis, Sara. *Sara's Story*. DVD

supplements (primarily from plants)

Di Paola, Robert S., M.D., and Timothy Grover. *A Doctor's Guide to Herbs and Supplements*

Gurudas, (much of this volume has been channeled through Jon C. Fox from Hilarion). *The Spiritual Properties of Herbs*

Heline, Corinne. *Magic Gardens*

McKenna, John, M.D. *Natural Alternatives to Antibiotics*

Murray, Michael T., N.D. *The Encyclopedia of Nutritional Supplements*

- - - . *Natural Alternatives to Over-the-Counter and Prescription Drugs*

Murray, Michael T., N.D., and Joseph Pizzorno, with Lara Pizzorno. *The Encyclopedia of Healing Foods*

Pelton, Ross, and Taffy Clarke Pelton. *Mind Food and Smart Pills*

Tenney, Louise. *Today's Herbal Health: The Essential Reference Guide*

Tierra, Michael, O.M.D. *Planetary Herbology: An Integration of Western Herbs Into the Traditional Chinese and Ayurvedic Systems*

White, Linda B., M.D., and Sharon Foster. *The Herbal Drugstore*

Williams, Jude C., M.H. *Jude's Herbal Home Remedies*

Wood, Matthew, Registered Herbalist. *The Book of Herbal Wisdom: Using Plants as Medicine*

alternative modalities

Andrews, Ted. *The Healing Manual: A Beginners Guide to Energy Therapies*

Bach, Edward, M.D. *Heal Thyself: An Explanation of the Real Cause and the Cure of Disease*

- - - . *The Twelve Healers and Other Remedies*

Baldwin, William J., D.D.S, Ph.D., Rev. *Spirit Releasement Therapy: A Technical Manual*

Bodine, Echo. *Hands That Heal*

Bradford, Michael, Intuitive Healer. *The Healing Energy of Your Hands*

Childre, Doc, Howard Martin, and Donna Beach. *The HeartMath® Solution*

Childre, Doc, and Deborah Rozman, Ph.D. *Transforming Stress: The HeartMath® Solution for Relieving Worry, Fatigue, and Tension*

supplementary readings and visuals

Craydon, Deborah, C.F.E.P., and Warren Bellows, Lic. Ac. *Floral Acupuncture: Applying the Flower Essences of Dr. Bach to Acupuncture Sites*

Dale, Cyndi. *New Chakra Healing: The Revolutionary 32-Center Energy System*

Detzler, Robert E. *Soul Re-Creation*

Devi, Lila. *The Essential Flower Essence Handbook*

Gordon, Richard. *Quantum Touch*

Griffin, Judy. *Flowers That Heal*

Gurudas. *Flower Essences and Vibrational Healing*

- - - . *Gem Elixirs and Vibrational Healing Vol. 1*

- - - . *Gem Elixirs and Vibrational Healing Vol. 2*

Heline, Corinne. *Healing and Regeneration Through Colour*

Hilarion, transmitted through Maurice B. Cooke. *Faces: Reading the Divine Analogy*

- - - , transmitted through Maurice B. Cooke. *Wildflowers: Their Occult Gifts*

Jell, Andreas. *Healing with Tachyon*

Krämer, Dietmar, Innovative Bach Flower Practitioner, with Helmut Wild. *New Bach Flower Body Maps: Treatment by Topical Application*

Millman, Dan. *The Life You Were Born To Live: A Guide to Finding Your Life's Purpose*

Pearl, Eric, D.C. *The Reconnection: Heal Others, Heal Youself*

Rand, William Lee. *Reiki for a New Millenium*

Rubenfeld, Fred, and Michael Smulkis. *Starlight Elixirs and Cosmic Vibrational Healing*

Sanders, Pete A. Jr. *You Are Psychic!: The Free Soul Method*

Shepard, Dr. Dorothy. *A Physician's Posy*

Tansley, David V., D.C. *Dimensions of Radionics*

- - - . *Radionics and the Subtle Anatomy of Man*

Targ, Russell. *The Limitless Mind: A Guide to Remote Viewing and Transformation of Consciousness*

- - - . *Miracles of Mind: Exploring Non-Local Consciousness and Spiritual Healing*

Thayer, Stevan J. *The Healing Angels of the Energy Fields*

Wauters, Ambika. *Homeopathic Colour Remedies*

gems and crystals

Ahsian, Naisha. *The Crystal Ally Cards: The Crystal Path to Self Knowledge*

- - - . *The Crystal Ally Cards.* the Cards

Bourgault, Luc (Blue Eagle). *American Indian Secrets of Crystal Healing*

Dolfyn. *Crystal Wisdom: Spiritual Properties of Crystals and Gemstones*

Melody. *Love is in the Earth: A Kaleidoscope of Crystals*

Raphael, Katrina. *Crystal Enlightenment: The Transforming Properties of Crystals and Healing Stones (Crystal Trilogy, Vol. 1)*

- - - . *Crystal Healing: Applying the Therapeutic Properties of Crystals and Stones (Crystal Trilogy, Vol. 2)*

- - - . *The Crystalline Transmission: A Synthesis of Light (Crystal Trilogy, Vol. 3)*

Roeder, Dorothy, channeled by. *Crystal Co-Creators*

Smith, Michael G. *Crystal Power*

dowsing

Gandrup, Robert. *Dowsing As a Daily Tool*

Korn, Joseph. *Dowsing: A Path to Enlightenment*

Nielsen, Greg, and Joseph Polansky. *Pendulum Power*

Paris, Don. *Regaining Wholeness Through the Subtle Dimensions: Where Science Meets Magic*

Schultz, David Allen. *Improve Your Life Through Dowsing*

Woods, Walt. *Letter to Robin: A Mini Course in Pendulum Dowsing*

runes

Blum, Ralph H. *The Book of Runes*

Pennick, Nigel. *The Complete Illustrated Guide to Runes: How to Interpret the Ancient Wisdom of the Runes*

Thorsson, Edred. *Runecaster's Handbook: The Well of Wyrd*

numerology

Dodge, Ellin. *Numerology Has Your Number*

Heline, Corinne. *The Sacred Science of Numbers*

Jordan, Juno. *Numerology: The Romance in Your Name*

Virtue, Doreen. *Angel Numbers 101*

music

Andrews, Ted. *Sacred Sounds*

Beaulieu, John, N.D., Ph.D. *Music and Sound in the Healing Arts: An Energy Approach*

Bentov, Itzhak. *Stalking the Wild Pendulum: On the Mechanics of Consciousness*

Berendt, Joachim-Ernst. *Nada Brahma, the World is Sound: Music and the Landscape of Consciousness*

- - - . *The Third Ear*

Bonny, Helen L., and Louis M. Savary. *Music and Your Mind: Listening with a New Consciousness*

Campbell, Don G. *Introduction to the Musical Brain*

- - - . *The Mozart Effect: Tapping the Powers of Music to Heal the Body, Strengthen the Mind, and Unlock the Creative Spirit*

- - - , compiled by. *Music and Miracles*

- - - . *The Roar of Silence: Healing Powers of Breath, Tone and Music*

Cook, Pat Moffitt, Ph.D., CCMHP. *The Open Ear Journals: Guide to Music and Healing*

Cousto, Hans, Mathematician and Musicologist. *The Cosmic Octave: Origin of Harmony, Planets, Tones, Colors, the Power of Inherent Vibrations*

David, William. *Harmonics of Sound, Colour and Vibration*

Dewhurst-Maddock, Olivea. *The Book of Sound Therapy: Heal Yourself with Music and Voice*

Eger, Joseph. *Einstein's Violin: A Conductor's Notes on Music, Physics, and Social Change*

Gardner, Kay, Teacher and Composer. *Sounding the Inner Landscape: Music as Medicine*

Garfield, Leah Maggie. *Sound Medicine*

Godwin, Joscelyn, Ph.D. (Musicology), ed. *Cosmic Music, Musical Keys to the Interpretation of Reality: Essays by Marius Schneider, Rudolf Haase, Hans Erhard Lauer*

- - - . *The Mystery of the Seven Vowels: In Theory and Practice*

Goldman, Jonathan. *Healing Sounds: The Power of Harmonics*

Hamel, Peter Michael. *Through Music to the Self: How to Appreciate and Experience Music Anew*

Heline, Corinne. *Beethoven's Nine Symphonies Correlated with the Nine Spiritual Mysteries*

- - - . *Color and Music in the New Age*

- - - . *The Cosmic Harp*

- - - . *The Esoteric Music of Richard Wagner*

- - - . *Healing and Regeneration Through Music*

- - - . *Music: The Keynote of Human Evolution*

Hodson, Geoffrey. *Music Forms: Superphysical Effects of Music Clairvoyantly Observed*

Hunt, Roland. *Fragrant and Radiant Healing Symphony: Colour, Sound, Perfume*

Kahn, Hazrat Inayat, Sufi Teacher. *The Music of Life*

Lingerman, Hal A. *The Healing Energies of Music*

McClellan, Randall, Ph.D. *The Healing Forces of Music*

Ristad, Eloise. *A Soprano on Her Head: Right-Side-Up Reflections on Life and Other Performances*

Rudhyar, Dane. *The Magic of Tones and the Art of Music*

Sacks, Oliver, M.D., Neurologist. *Musicophilia: Tales of Music and the Brain*

- - - . *Seeing Voices*

Scott, Cyril. *Music, Its Secret Influences Through the Ages*

Steindl-Rast, Brother David, Ph.D., Sharon Lebell, and Catholic Church Chant. *The Music of Silence: Entering the Sacred Rhythms of Monastic Experience*

Steindl-Rast, Brother David, Ph.D., and Sharon Lebell. *The Music of Silence: Entering the Sacred Space of Monastic Experience*

- - - . *The Music of Silence 2 Ed.: A Sacred Journey Through the Hours of the Day*

Steiner, Rudolf, Ph.D. (Philosophy). *The Inner Nature of Music and the Experience of Tone*

Stewart, R.J. *Music and the Elemental Psyche*

Tame, David. *The Secret Power of Music: The Transformation of Self and Society Through Musical Energy*

Wilson, Frank R. *Tone Deaf and All Thumbs: An Introduction to Music-Making*

aromatherapy

Balz, Rudolph. *The Healing Power of Essential Oils*

Catty, Suzanne. *Hydrosols: The Next Aromatherapy*

Cunningham, Scott. *Magical Aromatherapy: The Power of Scent*

Damian, Kate, and Peter Damian. *Aromatherapy: Scent and Psyche: Using Essential Oils for Physical and Emotional Well-Being*

Davis, Patricia. *Aromatherapy: An A-Z*

- - - . *Subtle Aromatherapy*

Lawless, Julia. *Aromatherapy and the Mind: The Psychological and Emotional Effects of Essential Oils*

Mailhebiau, Philippe. *Portraits in Oils: The Personality of Aromatherapy Oils and Their Link with Human Temperaments*

Mojay, Gabriel. *Aromatherapy for Healing the Spirit: Restoring Emotional and Mental Balance with Essential Oils*

Rose, Jeanne. *The Aromatherapy Book*

Schnaubelt, Kurt, Ph.D. (Chemistry). *Medical Aromatherapy: Healing with Essential Oils*

Tisserand, Maggie. *Aromatherapy for Women*

Valnet, Jean, M.D. *The Practice of Aromatherapy: A Classic Compendium of Plant Medicines and Their Healing Properties*

Winter, Ruth. *A Consumer's Dictionary of Cosmetic Ingredients*

Worwood, Valerie Ann. *The Fragrant Heavens, the Spiritual Dimension of Fragrance and Aromatherapy*

- - - . *The Fragrant Mind: Aromatherapy for Personality, Mind, Mood and Emotion*

part the sixth:
_____

showcasing the future

*affirming simplicity and the grace of
conciousness in expansion*

showcasing the future

publications

Bridges Magazine, the magazine of ISSSEEM — The International Society for the Study of Subtle Energies and Energy Medicine. www.issseem.org

Erowid Extracts, documenting the complex relationship between humans and psychoactives. www.erowid.org

The Maps Bulletin (MAPS — an acronym for Multidisciplinary Association for Psychedelic Studies). www.maps.org. Phone: 831-429-6362

The Noetic Post, a Bulletin from the Institute of Noetic Sciences, www.noetic.org

Shift, at the Frontiers of Consciousness, the Institute of Noetic Sciences Magazine. www.shiftinaction.com

future focused organizations

The Academy for Future Science, a non-profit corporation examining new scientific ideas for the future with an intention to enhance humanity's future creativity. P.O. Box FE, Los Gatos, CA. 95031. affs@affs.org

The Institute of HeartMath®, empowers heart-based living. founder, Doc Childre. www.heartmath.com

The Institute of Noetic Sciences. www.noetic.org

The International Society for the Study of Subtle Energies and Energy Medicine, "promotes understanding, exploration, reaseach, and application of the energies of consciousness."[1] www.issseem.org

The Living Essence Foundation, "exists to celebrate and to support this shift in global consciousness from separation to oneness."[2] original founder, Arjuna Ardagh. www.livingessence.com

The Multidisciplinary Association for Psychedelic Studies. www.maps.org

The New Age Bible and Philosophy Center, "a temple of ESOTERIC learning of the BIBLE, PHILOSOPHY, and other inspired teachings that are helpful and necessary for the advancement into the Acquarian Age."[3] a non-profit organization founded in 1931. Phone: 310-395-4346. Email: nabc@earthlink.net

---

[1] Quoted from an email from ISSSEEM April 20, 2010.
[2] Quoted from a Living Essence Foundation entry on the internet.
[3] Quoted from a New Age Bible and Philosophy Center brochure.

about the author

Patricia holds an undergraduate degree in philosophy from Wellesley and did subsequent studies in the psychology of space in the School of Architecture at M.I.T. In the last ten years she has applied herself to alternative understandings as they apply to health and to healing. She is drawn especially by the discipline's embrace of the soul and the soul's intimate relationship with the health of its corporeal vessel and by its understanding of the being as holistic rather than mechanistic.

Patricia received her ordination from the Lively Stones World Healing Fellowship under the tutelage of Willard Fuller, Th.D. The curriculum offered a fluid and non-denominational embrace of Christian doctrine in tandem with the esoteric realities of fields and energies and a lovely variety of quantum wisdoms paralleling ancient ones.

Patricia also trained at Hanna Kroeger's Peaceful Meadow Retreat in Boulder, Colorado and studied at the New Mexico School of Natural Therapeutics in Albuquerque. She studied acupressure privately with Norman Davies, protégé of (Doc) Fred Houston, D.C., D.D., Ph.D., and received his letter of commendation and acknowledgement of practice hours and studies completed. She is trained in Malcolm Rae's methods of subtle energy analysis, better known as radionics, trained as well in the use of flower and gem essences, and as a student of aromatherapy, has pursued advanced studies in the French method of layering the oils. For some time, the core of her hands-on work centered around Robert Detzler's spiritual response therapy (better known as SRT). A dowser for years, she found this work naturally inviting and watched it serve her energetically ultra-sensitive and equally energetically-compromised husband. Now in her sixth decade she decides to devote herself to the sacred opportunities of writing and of introducing the curious to pathways of initiation and study as they unfold themselves across the templates of their respective journeys.

Patricia's next work is in process — a trilogy exploring conscious death and dying and the reinvention of ourselves and our lives in the aftermath of a spouse's transition.

notes

www.ingramcontent.com/pod-product-compliance
Lightning Source LLC
Chambersburg PA
CBHW080239170426
43192CB00014BA/2494